THE CARE OF GIVING
FAMILY-IN-HOME CAREGIVING

JEAN RENEE PORTER

Self-Published: December 2017

Acknowledgments

First and foremost, I give thanks, praise and all glory to my Lord and Savior Jesus Christ for all he's done, doing and going to do. I have so much to be thankful for. Thank you for being the caregiver's caregiver, a way-maker, always making a way out of no way and while I'm trying to figure it out, you have already worked it out. Thank you for allowing me to fly solo, be home alone but not lonely, giving me the strength to live and enjoy life independently. Thank you for favoring me, surrounding me with so many earth angels, blessing me abundantly with good health and the ability to care for others. Thank you for making me a confident, intelligent and talented authoress-preneur. Thank you for teaching me that Jesus is the key to life and the way to an intimate relationship with You—God who holds the key to the path that leads to unraveling and unlocking mysteries and overcoming obstacles in life. Most importantly, thank you for teaching me that Thanksgiving is every day of my life, that failure to forgive affects me, in this life, and in the next, and that everyone must walk across the bridge of forgiveness if we are a true believer. Thank you for the anointing that you have bestowed upon me. I am Godspoiled and I have an attitude of gratitude.

I will sing unto the Lord, because he has been so good to me.
Psalm 13:6

Robin Fabrega – "We have the same Father"—your words. I touch and agree – we have the DNA of the Holy Spirit. God has given us the Holy Spirit to fill our hearts with His love. God is truly awesome. He knew long before we did that you would lose your mother and I would lose my husband therefore it was by design, miraculous intervention and divine placement orchestrated by God that brought you to California. Robin had never met Rick before then. Thank you for everything, I appreciate your prayers, sense of humor, encouragement, time, energy, silliness, and for being there when we really needed you because many will say they are your friend, but they are nowhere to be found when you really need one?

Most men will proclaim each his own goodness, but who can find a faithful man [friend]? Proverbs 20:6

Sister Fermer Rutherford, Word of Life Fellowship Center. Thank you for being a prayer warrior and keeping my family strong, protected and prayerful. Your actions clearly reflect your sanctity, admiration and love for our Lord. Your godliness kept Rick and I inspired during some very difficult, dark and uncertain times. You are a rarity, a saint, and a true child/friend of the King.

He that loveth pureness of heart, for the grace of his lips the King shall be his friend. Proverbs 22:11

Thank you, Pastor Kephyan Sheppard, who I met when he was an Elder at Family of Love Church. He is now the Pastor at Word of Life Fellowship Center. I sincerely appreciate you officiating Mr. Porter's memorial service with your uplifting, spiritual, motivational, and moving message, "What will your dash look like when you expire?" It was an amazing, thought-provoking, faith-lifting and inspirational homegoing service. Thank you for keeping us strong and encouraged with your steadfast ministry. Thank you for being such a good young pastor and our friend.

Is any sick among you? Let him call for the elders of the church; and let them pray over him, anointing him with oil in the name of the Lord: And the prayer of faith shall save the sick, and the Lord shall raise him up; and if he has committed sins, they shall have forgiven him. James 5:14-15

Cathy Jackson, Family of Love Church, thank you for the faith-lifts, your time, prayers, anointing, and blessons (blessings and lessons). Your prayers, faith, godliness and commitment to the Lord kept us grounded. You are living proof of God's miraculous healing powers. You endured it and you were delivered because you always believed that you would be, by the grace of God, you were, and you can see again. I admire your devoutness. You are an earth angel and my hero. I will forever remember you, who spoke the word of God to us. The amazing miracle of your sight returning was nothing but God. Thank you, God and thank you, Sister Cathy!

Remember them which have the rule over you, who have spoken unto you the word of God: whose faith follow, considering the end of their conversation. Hebrew 13:7

Bishop/Pastor James Young, Family of Love Church. Thank you for everything. I am so grateful and indebted to you for referring Pastor Sheppard. Thank you for taking the time out of your busy schedule to attend the memorial service, providing the food and all the other acts of generosity and graciousness that you and your various ministries extended to the Porter's. Thank you from the bottom of my heart for adopting the Porter's and welcoming them with open arms into the Family of Love Church.

The LORD is good, a strong hold in the day of trouble; and he knoweth them that trust in him. Nahum 1:7

Millie Jackson and daughter, Courtney, thanks for being my first Cali friends and for referring me to Family of Love Church. I love and appreciate you both. Millie, an amputee and heart attack survivor had her own health issues, but she was always in good spirits, cooking, making homemade candy, uplifting, helping and witnessing to others, including the Porter's.

Let us therefore make every effort to do what leads to peace and to mutual edification. Romans 14:19

Thank you to my sister Cheryl Freeland. I have an attitude of gratitude and I will always cherish you and remember your selfless act and generosity in providing me with my first laptop which seems like umpteen years ago. You gave me the boost and the main tool that I needed to make my dream a reality. I love you from infinity and beyond. I love and appreciate you, thanks, sis–I called her "daddy" although she takes after my mom too who taught us about having a tool box and household essentials, but Cheryl puts it to good use, the rest of us call a handyman. However, I loved assisting my dad with changing faucets, hanging ceiling fans and chandeliers, and other electrical fixtures, and repairing washing machines, he helped me to make a homemade lamp—I was his little helper and right-hand gal. My brother worked with him in between school but that was expected, Cheryl, on the hand was a bonus, a devoted daughter who made sacrifices to work at his laundry where people dropped off their clothes before work and picked them up after work. She believed strongly that God designed us to live in families and family relationships were very important.

Children are a gift from the Lord; they are a reward from him. Psalm 12:3

James "Toby" Johnson, Juan "Poone" Johnson, and Dana "Spunky" Tolson, my kids and my favorite people in the entire world – you are my bright light at the end of the tunnel. I love you for your encouragement, confidence, faith and unconditional love. Keep making mercy deposits by teaching your children that Jesus is the key to life so that they will teach their children, and their children will teach their children and so on – and you all will be rewarded with God's Benefit Package.   Thanks for all my grand and great grandchildren. I am a praying and super proud mama and granny. I love you all to eternity and beyond. You fill my life with joy, peace of mind, and a glad heart.

Correct thy son and he shall give thee rest; yea, he shall give delight unto thy soul. Proverbs 29:17

Ms. Bonnie Beck, Charter Hospice (Colton, CA) – Thank you, you were a Godsend. I learned a lot about hospice and appreciate all the information, help and support that you provided me, just in the nick of time, because the caregiver really needed a caregiver. My husband never got the hospice experience so although you had not technically started caring for him, you provided me with a sitter (on Friday and he passed away that Monday). Prior to that experience, I had no idea that hospice was the caregiver's caregiver or cared as much about the caregiver as the patient and that truly warmed my heart because I really needed someone to care about me and give me a break at that time, so thanks for stepping in and providing a sitter and relieving me, probably saving my life. I honestly felt that I could not go another day, and that is why I finally gave into hospice in the first place. I may not have made it until Monday myself had you not stepped in when you did. With all my love, thank you and God bless you and all the Charter Hospice earth angels.

Are they not all ministering spirits sent forth to minister for those who will inherit salvation? Hebrews 1:14

Nurse Danielle and CNA Maria, along with all the nurses, nurse assistants, aides and wound care specialist at Valu-Care Home Care Health Services (West Covina, CA) and

Desert Regional Hospital (Palm Springs, CA) – without you, I was lost. Thank you for your support, professionalism, expertise, guidance and tender loving care. Everyone had such ministering spirits and I am so happy and grateful to have been touched by you all. You were all God sent earth angels and a blessing to our lives.

Rejoice always, pray without ceasing, and in everything give thanks; for this is the will of God in Christ Jesus for you. 1 Thessalonians 5:16-18

DaVita Dialysis Center, an enormous thank you to Dr. Bartesé and his dialysis team of nutritionists, case workers, nurses and dialysis techs that were all-natural born angels, my heroes, as well as the greatest group of dedicated, compassionate and passionate people I've ever met. Dr. Bartesé, your bedside manners were beyond reproach. Thank you for always being available and super supportive. You were the absolute best and nicest doctor ever. We were very fortunate to have you on our team. Thank you!

For He shall give His angels charge over you, to keep you in all your ways. Psalm 91:11

John Grabb, thank you for making Mr. Porter the happiest sick man on earth once he was finally able to start peritoneal dialysis. It was something he wanted to do for a very long time – I regret that we did not start sooner. Thanks for the training, certification, patience and constant support. You have such a huge and giving heart. You made Rick feel special when he found a Redskin fan in Cali. I can never thank you enough and you have already earned your wings. Thanks for giving Mr. Porter your best, on so many levels— you were the best friend and nurse ever with your kind, caring, giving and loving ways.

We make a living by what we get. We make a life by what we give. Winston S. Churchill

Tanya Fowler, thank you so much for the love, faith-lifts, genuine friendship, concern, kindness, generosity and especially for being there for me every day, every step of the way from Virginia to California. You were good medicine for my soul, always having something positive, kind and godly to say. No one can break things down like you, little sis, Ms. Analytical. You are truly my sister in Christ. I love and appreciate you with all my heart. You are such a godly, generous and giving soul. I pray for good health, wealth, and that God blesses you with all your heart desires.

Beloved, I pray that you may prosper in all things and be in health, just as your soul prospers. 3 John 1:2

Ukali "Ukkie" Linda Bethea Wilson, thank you for introducing me to Khalil Gibran, Reiki and juicing 40 years ago. You have always been a natural dose of medicine in my life and a genuine friend, something that I will always cherish. You inspired me to be a life coach to others like you were to me. You and I have always had a spiritual connection. Also, you have always been an empowering, motivational and inspirational force in my life. I love you, David, and the family, everlastingly.

Generosity is giving more than you can, and pride is taking less than you need. Khalil Gibran

Dianne Camp, my longest and dearest friend, my ride or die. We had 60 years of friendship when you got your wings, and not everyone can say that they have had a friend for that many years. Our friendship was ordained by God and His divine placement and He makes no mistakes. A friendship like ours is a rarity. My life will never be the same without you. I thank you and your family for entrusting you into my care. It was just what we needed before you parted this earth. We had some hilarious and glorious times together, reading the bible, praying, eating, laughing, fun times with your children, grandchildren, family and friends. It takes a lot of time to develop a friendship like ours. Casual friends are plentiful but genuine friends are very few. You were a true "BFF", a priceless gift from God, your friendship and love compares to none other, it cannot be exchanged or replaced by money or for payment of any kind and you were a gift, a precious gem and I miss you greatly. Even when we didn't see each other or talk, that friendship and love was still there, and we could always pick up where we left off. When you were present in the body, I used to say, "I love you to life," now, "I love you to death." I keep shaking my head and repeating, "Absent in the body, present with the Lord." Rest in Paradise, my friend, my angel.

A good friend knows everything about you. A best friend has lived through everything with you.

Angie and Brian Spedden are my fungal (fun gal) and fungi (fun guy). They love to be threatened with a good time. "I be white black" and "I be white here" was how Brian and I poked fun at each other. You were the best friends and neighbors. You are my BFE (Best Friends Ever) and I have infinite love for you two. I could not have survived caregiving without you two. They were a Godsend and the caregiver's caregiver too because they took care of Rick and me. Everyone comes into your life for a reason or a season. You were our backbones, literally. Rick adored and loved you guys. I will always love and appreciate you. You have a genuinely caring, giving and loving nature. Everybody needs the Spedden's in their life. Thanks for being there for us and allowing me to lean on you whenever I needed a shoulder, hug, drink or escape. You are framily! Love & Happiness!

Genuine friends are powerful people; they are like family, they set well with your soul, good medicine for the spirit, dependable, and the best support system ever.

Danita Rudisill is my New York connection. A friend sharpens and refines a friend. Thank you for the endless acts of kindness you have done over the years, including lending me a desk top and laptop computers to get my writing started before I had my own computer. Your generosity to provide me with the means to type and put my books in motion was a huge contribution to me becoming the self-published authoress-preneur I am today. You have been a true friend and blessing in my life for 25 years. I love and appreciate you, thank you for all that you do from the heart. You are a true friend and a cheerful giver! I love you with all my heart and soul.

Iron sharpeneth iron, so a friend sharpens a friend. Proverbs 27:17

To my BFFs, Jesse Thompkins, Edith Burkett, Joanne Morrison, Brenda Mitchell, Thomasine Cox and Brenda Marshall: There are only three words for y'all, "I LOVE YOU!" I cherish our over 50-years of friendship and if I were to have my heart examined, there would be a picture of you embedded deep in my heart.

Best friends are like stars on a cloudy night, you may not see them, but they are always there, through thick and thin, their friendship will shine through. John Gabriel

Finally, my siblings, Dr. Larry Washington (Denalia), Cynthia Newman, Cheryl Freeland (Moochie), Terry

Washington and Keith Washington (Michelle) – God has been good to us, we are Godspoiled! I love and appreciate you to life. My best friends start with you, my framily! May God continue to bless you and yours.

A new commandment I give to you, that you love one another; as I have loved you, that you also love one another. John 13:34

Dedications

This book is dedicated to the 40 million heroes and heroines who sacrifice their jobs, family, time, energy and life to care for a disabled, chronically or terminally ill loved one or patient from an infant to the elderly. Caregiving is very challenging, testing, and demanding. Caregiving can take a toll on your health, emotionally and physically, your family life, and all your relationships. Caregivers seldom get to enjoy the fruits of their labors and the sad thing is that our society does not value the disabled, terminally ill, or elderly enough to provide adequate support or caregiving to them, so I am hopeful that the future brings more awareness to caregivers' increasing demand as well as the training, tools and support needed to provide the best, most affordable, safest, and healthiest family-in-home caregiving experience possible. Families need all the help they can get with keeping their loved ones at home rather than in a home.

Now hope does not disappoint, because the love of God has been poured out in our hearts by the Holy Spirit who was given to us. Romans 5:5

This book was inspired by my best friend, my angel, my dear and beloved late husband, Ricardo Porter, Sr. (02/07/54-11/14/11) – Gone much too soon but God knows best and He makes no mistakes. You taught me what unconditional love truly is. Death ends a life, not a relationship. Our love was strong, you will always live in my heart and be the love of my life. Memories are forever. Rest in Paradise, my love.

Wives, submit to your own husbands, as to the Lord. Ephesians 5:22

My Aunt Colleen Thorpe, got her wings at the age of 87 years young. She was the first caregiver that I ever knew.

She took care of everyone from foster children to the elderly, including babysitting for family and neighborhood kids. She was a phenomenal woman, an advocate for children; she was a household name in the community, involved with the civic association and the county public school system. She spent much of her life doing for others. I am so grateful to her for being a part of the village that raised me. She pierced my ears and coordinated with my mother to do my hair when my mother couldn't do it when I was young. I will always treasure the summers and New Year's Day family reunions we celebrated at her house all my life. "God is a just God," are her famous words to me. You are deeply missed, Auntie. Thank God for teaching me about caregiving, service and missionary work; all the blessons, stories, family history, pictures, time and good memories we shared. I will cherish our quality time together and our talks about God, family and love. We had some good times, just you and me, OG. I miss you sorely! Tears! Rest in Paradise, Auntie.

Service to others is the rent you pay for your room here on earth. Muhammad Ali

Paula Buckner is my cousin who is more like a big sister. We have always shared a very special bond growing up, and we have always been inseparable. Being the oldest, she looked after her many foster siblings, her younger siblings and cousins like me. Paula's door was always opened to anyone needing a home. Cuz, you are living proof that it's never too late to fulfill your dreams. You should be proud of all your accomplishments. Thank you for being my big cousin-sister-friend, and my ride or die. Continue to live the life you love and love the life you live. You are blessed to be in good health and still working so keep the faith and keep serving the Lord because nothing compares to God's Benefits Package.

Blessed be the Lord, who daily loads us with benefits, the God of our salvation! Psalm 68:19

Table of Contents

Introduction

This book is about a family in-home caregiving experience from beginning to end, inspired by the authoress' caregiving of her terminally ill husband for many years. It expresses how she felt, what she went through, what she did to survive it, and some tools she learned along the way. Ms. Porter said, "It was 'the care of giving' orchestrated by God (the caregiver's caregiver) that really got me through it and I cannot reiterate enough that I found peace, patience, strength, comfort, love and everything that I needed, in the bible. God surrounded me with quite a few earth angels. He does work in mysterious and miraculous ways. Not that I didn't get frustrated or wasn't faced with many difficult challenges, but God's word gave me endurance and it kept me in stride despite the difficult times and feelings of despair, darkness and uncertainty."

For there are three that bear record in heaven, the Father, the Word, and the Holy Ghost: and these three are one. 1 John 5:7

"The Care of Giving" is all about the caregiving process and is for everyone because life can change in an instant and the face of caregiving has changed considerably over the years. Unfortunately, there are just as many young people as elderly people disabled and needing constant care. Trying to care for a loved one at home who is disabled, chronically or terminally ill is not easy and it is normal for every caregiver to become discouraged and feel overwhelmed. In addition, it has become more difficult and demanding to care for a loved one because nowadays you must know as much as a nurse since the hospital stays are shorter due to costs, budget cuts, insurance, including the uninsured and underinsured. Unfortunately, caregivers do not have the training, skills, tools, benefits, incentives, days off, or pay that nurses have so they are already at a great disadvantage therefore it becomes the responsibility of the family. God is the caregiver's caregiver, so he will help you and your family get through anything, since you are adopted into God's family and members of His family too.

Now therefore ye are no more strangers and foreigners, but fellow citizens with the saints, and of the household of God. Ephesians 2:19

It takes everything you got to be a caregiver including even temperament, endurance, prayers, patience, survival skills, tenacity, toughness, guts, courage, self-control, advocacy, kindness, pure heartedness, open-mindedness, gratitude, love, honesty, encouragement, respect, thoughtfulness, and most of all, the love of God and the only real incentive or motivation that caregivers have is their faith, patience, love and good heartedness. Thank God for all the earth angels God sent to help us.

Giving is motivated by loving and love is the one thing we can spread around and not run out of so start a love epidemic, overdose on love. Love is what we all need more of.

The authoress is hopeful that *"The Care of Giving"* will provide the guidance, education, skills, tools and awareness to the labor of caregivers since they are not alone. She shares her true story to give the full picture of the caregiving

2

process and the many challenges one may face along their caregiving journey.   Every caregiving experience is different, some worse than others but it all depends on the illness and the family's support system.

Chapter 1

Love at First Date

Rick and I first met over the phone by way of my niece Shawn and after speaking to him for several hours we decided to set a blind date. I was looking forward to meeting him especially since his best friend, James, and his girlfriend and my niece's best friend, Eudora were all playing cupid. All of them had already pumped the both of us up about the other. They had been trying for a long time to hook us up, but I had been dragging my feet since I was in a five-year stagnant relationship with Nick. We were basically finished years ago but out of habit and attachment he was an itch I couldn't get rid of but as soon as I set the date with Rick I broke it off with Nick and told him he was no longer welcomed to come by my home, unannounced anymore. He threatened to come by anyway, any time he pleased but he was no fool and after a few weeks passed without seeing him or hearing from him, I figured the coast was clear. Out with old, and in with the new. I prayed Nick away and God answered my prayers. Praise the Lord. He was finally gone. That was a blessing. I was feeling blessed.

But I know that when I come to you, I shall come in the fullness of the blessing of the gospel of Christ. Romans 15:29

Now that Rick's birthday and Valentine's Day were out of the way, we decided to get together. He picked me up from work in DC. He had a very nice forest green Nissan Frontier pick-up truck and when he got out of the truck to open my door, I noticed the brother was cleaner than the board of health, suited down, a gentleman, and he was handsome too. There was an instant attraction. He greeted me with a dozen

1

of dark purple roses, something I have never seen before, so I was very curious and anxious to find out what purple roses meant. I didn't have to wonder too long. "Purple roses represent magic and charm," he explained, "it's an expression of love at first date." I think he made that up, but purple was my favorite color and they were gorgeous, so it really didn't matter. On top of the to-die-for roses, he also gave me an expensive bottle of Founders Reserve Pinot Noir and a box of chocolate candy filled with caramel, all my favorites. Plus, he had me smiling from ear to ear. He greeted me with a tight hug and he smelled so good I could have sniffed him all night and I was allergic to most colognes. So that he could drive, he handed me a newspaper so that I could find out what time the movie started that he had chosen since I had not been to the movies in over 10 years and had no idea what movie we should see. We had also previously planned to go out to dinner, but he had already done so much for me that I was dying to do something nice for him as well. I invited him to my place for dinner before going to the movies. I wanted to change my clothes, and being a Friday night, my oldest son was cooking fried fish, steamed shrimp, homemade macaroni and cheese, fresh veggie salad and broccoli. "My son is the bomb cook," I said, "he cooks like me, with a lot of love." He joked about looking forward to meeting his future son-in-law. I liked him a lot. I was enjoying his company immensely. My son was also a mixologist at the Washington Hotel, The Venetian, and frequently bartender at hundreds of private events and banquets in the DC area and out of town. He and I also did catering on the side. In addition, he was the manager at the historical Watergate Restaurant in Washington, D.C. so he was no stranger when it came to hospitality; he was Mr. Hospitable himself. He was the host with the most. He served Rick a virgin drink and me an extra dry Martini with extra olives. Rick enjoyed everything and was quite impressed with my son's cooking abilities because

2

the young man knew his way around the kitchen and he had good presentation. I was used to it and wouldn't expect anything less, but I was very appreciative and so was Rick, it saved him some money too because I am not a cheap date. We talked about everything: family, mother, father, kids, exes, and life, in general. He voluntarily shared, "I have two kids, a girl and boy, a stepdaughter and one granddaughter, my stepdaughter's child. I hate the word 'step' and 'half', but it is, what it is. I've been married twice, I love being married and I'll do it again and again until I get it right, I'm a diabetic, I have two sisters and three brothers, and both parents are deceased, I work at the university and I used to work at the hospital. I am a native Washingtonian; I got property in Orange, Virginia, and an apartment in DC." He was an open book, very honest, easy going, transparent, even-tempered, and a good guy. Thank God, he wasn't a drinker, drunk, drug addict, drug dealer or jailbird. I began talking about my children nonstop. We both had three children and his youngest child, and I shared the same name; and he, his son and my youngest son shared the same name. We both felt that was more than just a coincidence. He was choking up as he spoke lovingly and highly of his mother, how he took care of her prior to her passing, and how much he loved and missed her. His mother was an only child, born with one kidney. She was among the first black head nurses at a prominent hospital in DC back in the 50s. I adored a man who loves and respects his mother. He loved his grandparents too who he was privileged to grow up with in the same household. His grandfather was a Mason and a Deacon at the church. Their pastor frequently visited their home, practically every Sunday for dinner. Rick attended Catholic school and graduated from an all-male public vocational high school. We both smiled as we walked and talked and passed time getting acquainted while waiting for the movie to start. For someone who first appeared very quiet and reserved, now had plenty to say. We talked nonstop. The date wasn't even over yet, it had just begun, and I was already anticipating a second date. Kudos to all the cupids. The movie "Civil Action" with John Travolta was about water contamination. It was an amazing, educational and quite relevant movie at that time and for many years to come. By the end of the night we were best friends forever. We were behaving like teens, butterflies, blushing, hugging and kissing like we've known each other all our lies. He said it was love at first date, but for me, he was too good to be true. He was quiet with a sweet, kind-hearted, and loving demeanor. I did not want this night to end. I was on cloud nine, literally. Life was good, I wasn't looking for a boyfriend but it looks like a boyfriend found me, and he was amazing, a Godsend. God is good. Whoever pursues godliness will find it.

He who follows righteousness and mercy finds life, righteousness, and honor. Proverbs 21:21

Although I wasn't looking for a serious relationship I had a feeling that he was the one, that he was that man I had been waiting and praying for. The way that he smiled and looked at me gave me the impression that the attraction was mutual. He was so different than all the other guys I had dated. I felt I had known him forever. He was stable, self-sufficient, serious, and he had a good sense of humor. I was falling in love. He was way different than "can't get right" Nick. I was so ready to move on. I was tired of wasting my time, being nice, settling for less and considering everyone else's feelings but mine. Rick called me Mother Teresa. I was no Mother Teresa, I was just a goodhearted woman, no one special, a giver. Rick had me forgetting all about Nick. Good riddance! When I first met Nick, we were inseparable, and I thought he had a lot of potential but in time he proved that he didn't have anything to bring to the table but an appetite. He did have a job, but it didn't pay much, and he was always making repairs to his used beat up cars, his life was plagued with constant issues with broken down cars. He wasn't doing anything but taking up space. I was cordial to Nick, but it was getting harder and harder to ignore and accept his freeloading, immature, irritating, leeching, attitude. Enough is enough.

Kindness is in our power, even when fondness is not. Samuel Johnson

Moving Forward

Rick was truly a breath of fresh air in my life. He had that wow factor and he literally swept me off my feet. He loved to travel, and he had his own money. He was very practical and frugal. He dressed to impress. He had property, an apartment, and a reliable vehicle, a permanent job with benefits and good tenure. I had helped so many men in my lifetime. He didn't mind spending his money and he was all about pleasing me. Hanging out with Rick was like hanging out with one of my girls; he liked to do whatever I wanted to do so I would hang out with him any day. He loved sex, but it did not define our relationship. He was the best thing that had ever happened to me. Rick met most of my ideal man qualities and criteria. He had a sweet spirit; he was passionate, compassionate, strong, caring, positive, creative, understanding, trustworthy, affectionate, kind, loving, romantic, charming, personable, gainfully employed, and a good communicator. He was special, and I could see myself with him down the road and for a very long time. As a matter of fact, I was so comfortable with him that I shared with him my passion and dream to write a book, and that one day I would be an author-preneur, I had tons of journals, notebooks and pads filled with years of my writings, but I just could never find the time to type them up. He was super impressed and said, "I know a lot of people who said they wanted to write a book, but I've never known anyone who has actually written one, we must bring that dream to life. You could be my very first 'authoress-preneur' friend." I was smiling and filled with excitement. "Authoress-preneur, I really like the sound of that," I said, "I just need to type and publish them first." After going out for a month, he called my bluff, told me to pack several days of clothes, and my journals because he was taking me away for the long weekend to get my authoress-preneur on. I was excited but there was only one problem, neither of us had a laptop or desktop computer and I was borrowing my girlfriend Danita's desktop computer as it was. He had no need or desire for a computer. I called Danita to tell her my opportunity and dilemma because I thought about taking her desktop with me, but she brought a laptop by for me to take instead. She was a lifesaver. He took me to a nice secluded quiet spot in the country, 65 miles from where I lived. He let me write and he would only disturb or interrupt me to eat the delectable meals he had prepared for my breaks and he was a darn good cook, quite impressive, crab cakes, fish, shrimp, home fries, cabbage, and coleslaw. I wrote until my heart was content from Friday night to Sunday morning. We went to my childhood church, lunch and home to prepare for the week. When I told him that going to church made my week go better, he started going every Sunday with me.

And on the seventh day God ended His work which He had done, and He rested on the seventh day from all His work which He had done. Genesis 2:2

He was so kind, easy, considerate and such a gentleman, always putting me first. Every weekend, we went somewhere, anywhere. We went to the Virgin Islands. We would even take a ride to Philly just to get a Philly cheesesteak and come right back in time for Sunday football. I loved Virginia Beach and Myrtle Beach while he loved Ocean City, Rehoboth, Dewey, and Bethany beaches. He was spoiling the heck out of me and no matter where we went he made sure that I had whatever my little heart desired. I never had anyone be happy just because I was happy. We were going places we had never been and seeing things we had never seen before. I loved the mountains and he loved the ocean, so we frequented places that had both views, we went paddle boarding, paddle boat riding and watched many sunrises, stars, and sunsets.

I made a lot of progress in no time flat with my first book. I organized my writings and was writing every chance I got, practically two-three hours a day. I was so grateful and indebted to him. He and I had gotten close fast. We were already talking about retirement which really wasn't that far off for me since I had always planned to retire at 55. He was two years younger than me and had plans to retire a couple years after me. He motivated and supported me. I felt productive. Consistently for about two years, every Friday, Rick would pick me up from work and take me away for the entire weekend and treat me like a queen. I had accomplished a lot with him and I was thankful to have him in my life. We would eat and drink and be merry every time I finished a new chapter. He inspired me and had me feeling extremely blessed.

I know that nothing is better for them than to rejoice, and to do good in their lives, and also that every man should eat and drink and enjoy the good of all his labor—it is the gift of God. Ecclesiastes 3:13

Suddenly, our getaway trips came to an abrupt halt. For over a year, I was given no explanation why, so I had no idea why Rick stopped taking me to the country and if I did not trust him I would have thought he was cheating on me. Finally, he told me that his son had come to him saying that his sister was being evicted and needed a place to stay, so he gave up his humble abode to his stepdaughter and her family. The only reason the subject came up in the first place was because he was complaining about her not paying the rent, paying late, and he had an issue with a returned check for insufficient funds that she was stopping by to make good on. He was furious because all he charged her was $650 a month for a three bedrooms with family room, living room, two bathrooms. Where else could she live for that? Some folks just can't be helped. "Plus, she has a husband," he added. It

8

amazed me how nice Rick was to his stepdaughter who had a real sense of entitlement. I told him that his daughter should be held accountable for her actions, but he would be blessed for his unselfishness, giving up his getaway to provide her ungrateful behind with a place for her and her family to stay. According to Rick, it wasn't the first time she had bounced a check, so I was disturbed and disappointed to hear that, but it was none of my business. I thought she was the one that would treat her father the best because he always spoke so highly of her and put her on a pedestal, but this chick had feet of clay. I hadn't met her yet and really didn't want to. She sounded self-destructive to me, but Rick said she had an irresponsible husband. He took up for her, everything was her husband's fault. I told him to stop talking about them because I wasn't going to like either of them when I do finally meet them.

But the mercy of the Lord is from everlasting to everlasting on those who fear Him, and His righteousness to children's children, too such as keep His covenant, and to those who remember His commandments to do them. Psalm 103-17-18

On my 50th birthday, we had a lot to celebrate. I published my first book; it was my birthday present to me. I felt a real since of pride and accomplishment thanks to Rick and my good friend Gail Cook who paid for my first self-published book. God bless her soul, and may she rest in paradise. Unfortunately, Gail's untimely death occurred when a 23-year-old hit her head-on and they both were killed. Rick and I celebrated for Gail too as we indulged in lobster salad, sesame noodles, caviar and champagne. She loved the good life, she wore nothing but linen and drove a Mercedes. She worked as a receptionist at a law firm and a funeral home part-time. She had planned to accompany Rick and me to my book events. I miss her immensely. Gail was one of my biggest fans. Absent from the body, present with the Lord.

The timeliness of death has nothing to do with age, rather it has everything to do with our relationship with God, who created us, and who has chosen the time to give us our wings.

Rick and I traveled a lot for my speaking engagements, awards, promoting and marketing my book. He loved attending my tea and wine times with the authoress, dinner parties, public speaking, book clubs, book signings, book conventions, conferences, dances, and any venues that I was invited to. He never missed an event no matter where it took us. We also found ourselves supporting other self-published authors as well. It was a very proud moment for me too because it was many years in the making and Rick was my biggest supporter and number one fan. He started the ball rolling and stood by me every step of the way. I love him for giving me the peacefulness, quietness, encouragement, motivation, and support that I needed all the way to the end to accomplish this mission. He was there for me, patient, calm, encouraging, loving, and when it was born, one would have thought that we had just delivered a healthy baby in our old age. He was so ecstatic he purchased a private stock of about 150 books that he sold from his truck wherever we went. Whenever I spoke or appeared he had his stock which meant I always had plenty of books on hand. He was too funny, and he was happier than I was. I loved that man for having that type of faith and confidence in me. He really was all about me, I had finally written my first book, and I couldn't be more excited or happier. I had a good man and I wrote a book. I was a beast! Right from the beginning, I knew Rick was the one. He had my heart. We were road dawgs and living the life of Riley. For years things were going hot and heavy between Rick and me. We were having a blast and living a blissful life. He often talked about marriage, but I always got off the subject because I was happy just the way things were. He had money, I had money, and together there were no limitations, we went for the gusto and we were always going places and doing fun stuff. Our life was magical, a real fairytale. I was not rushing marriage or planning on shacking up anytime soon. I was good.

Walked In, But Not Out

A little after our five-year anniversary, one gorgeous bright and sunny fall September day, Rick went to work as usual as a driver for the President's office in the transportation department at the local university where he had worked for approximately 15 years. By early afternoon, he was complaining about not feeling well. An hour or so later he was feeling worse, so he left work which was unusual for him. He made it home safely, took a shower and afterwards said that he felt light headed, "swimming in the head" as he described it. He then fell asleep. Several hours later he called me to say that he was unbalanced so I suggested he immediately take an aspirin which he did. He proceeded to get dressed, he left his apartment building, made it outside, climbed into his stick shift pick-up truck, and by the grace of God managed to drive himself all the way to the hospital, on the other side of town from southeast to northwest passing a couple of hospitals along the way. He arrived at the hospital safely and in one piece however his right hand and fingers were numb, so he was unable to sign his name. He was admitted immediately and placed under observation. There were no rooms available, so he was placed in the hallway outside the emergency room until a room became available and in the meantime, they would monitor him periodically and order any necessary tests, but they had absolutely no idea when he might get a room because they were just that overcrowded. As ridiculous as that may have sounded there was nothing that we could do about it because the hospital was full. He really did not appreciate being placed in the hallway overnight and he felt as an employee of the university and an ex-employee of the hospital, he deserved better treatment. We were both frustrated about not having a diagnosis and being left in the hallway indefinitely was not good for anyone's morale. After a couple of days, he had had enough of being surrounded by chaos, loud noises, people congregated in groups, odors, cursing, and serious emergencies happening all around him. He just couldn't rest or get comfortable in the hallway. I asked him to stop complaining because it could be worse, they could have turned him away, had him go someplace else but they didn't so be thankful for that, if nothing else. He adjusted his attitude somewhat and the complaining subsided a bit, but he honestly felt neglected and forgotten so he really thought if he were in a room he may get the attention he needed. He decided to call the President's assistant at the university. Within the hour, I was thrilled and shocked when he called to say he was in a private room. That was fast, and he sounded fantastic. He even told me to take my time getting to the hospital which was a relief since I had planned to visit him on my lunch hour, but my boss had other plans for my lunch hour. He was having lunch delivered to me, so at one point I was expected to be at the office, and at the hospital too. I sure couldn't be two places at once. In fairness to my boss, I was way too busy, he was in court, so I had to be in the office. I was also entitled to lunch, but I also had a partner, an associate, a paralegal, and clients all depending on me also for everything. This was business. I was a Girl Friday, the billing coordinator, office manager, legal assistant, researcher, travel agent and receptionist. Lawyers do not understand anything except catering to them and dollar signs. I not only worked through lunch, I came close to working through dinner, and I still hadn't gotten to the hospital to see Rick. They could have cared less, totally heartless and if I had left my work undone, they would have fired me. As far as they were concerned the only place that I needed to be was at work. That was beside the point, I wanted to be by Rick's side and he needed me to be there for moral support, if nothing else. I did not want him to be alone. When I was finally able to leave which was much later than I had planned, I called Rick to tell him that I was on my way and after being on the phone with him for about 15 seconds I heard an extremely loud thump and the phone went silent. It sounded like he hit the floor and I began to imagine the worse. I yelled his name repeatedly to the top of my lungs through the phone, but he didn't respond. I felt helpless because I knew Rick was in trouble. I used my cell phone to call the nurse's station. I asked the nurse who answered the phone to please go to Mr. Porter's room to check on him. I had not hung up the work landline that was on speaker at the time, so I could clearly hear every word the nurse spoke out of her mouth with her broken English, and heavy Nigerian accent when she entered his room and yelling, "Mr. Potta, Mr. Potta, who da yell told shoe to jit oudda da dom bed? Jit up, I was just hair tree minutes ago, you should've called, look wat you done to yousef?" Marking the nurse, Rick said, "Nah, you are a liar, eyes haven't seen you all moaning, at least tree ours, fer sher. No one ever came to check on me, or told me that I couldn't get oudda da dom bed eva. I had to use the bathroom, so I fell trying to use the dom bathroom and why the heck you talking to me like that anyway, who da yell you think you're talking to, lady?" Rick was sweet, but he was a no-nonsense person

14

who had zero tolerance for a liar. He was not confrontational, but he would defend himself. I was so relieved to hear his voice, but I was still concerned about why he fell (on the hospital's watch) in the first place, and of course I was praying for the best, but preparing myself for the worse. At least he was still alive. Maybe he was better off in the hallway. This was ludicrous. I rushed to the hospital and when I arrived I was informed that he had suffered an ischemic stroke, which left him with right-side weakness and he could have many more mini strokes. I could not believe my ears. He has been having a stroke for three days, obviously. I just couldn't stop shaking my head or figure out how this could have happened in the hospital. These people were making me lose my religion. What the fork? I was angry, crying, seeing blood and I could not understand how someone could come to the hospital with stroke-like symptoms, be under observation for several days and have a stroke that cripples him possibly for life, under their watch right before their very eyes, and shortly after he was placed in a room. I was in total disbelief and we both had lost all faith in that hospital. I wasn't that impressed as it was since they ran out of essentials: urinals, water pitchers, wash basins, and basic hygiene products, things they should never run out of. I was glad that they did not turn Rick away or refuse him treatment, but at the same time it is bad when the hospital starts placing patients in the hallway and forget all about them, no diagnosis, tests, lab work or prognosis and they have a stroke that possibly could have been avoided. I was irate, and the hospital had plenty of explaining to do. I felt they were very careless and extremely negligent. Rick had a serious stroke which affected the side of his brain that controlled his emotions, and right-side movement. He could have died so he was blessed to be alive, his mouth or body wasn't twisted, and his speech wasn't affected, but his arm was limp due to nerve damage that bothered him tremendously to the point where he referred to himself as afflicted and he was wheelchair bound. It was a lot to digest. Rejoice in hope, endure in sickness, determination and unwavering prayer. All I could say was, pray, pray, pray, every night and day.

Be kindly affectionate to one another with brotherly love, in honor giving preference to one another; not lagging in diligence, fervent in spirit, serving the Lord; rejoicing in hope, patient in tribulation, continuing steadfastly in prayer. Romans 12:10-12

Eight days later he was discharged from the hospital. His stepdaughter and son were there to pick us up. Bless their heart since they had driven from Virginia to DC. Rick's son drove his father's truck, and his daughter drove his son's vehicle from the hospital to my house. Sadly, Rick walked in, but he did not walk out. He was pushed out in a wheelchair. His children dropped us off at my place in Maryland and they went on their merry way. The very next morning, a Saturday, Rick and I were at the cardiologist, Dr. Collison's office near my home that was normally closed on the weekends, but opened just for Rick. Dr. Collison turned out to be one of the best cardiologists in his field. Rick's heart prognosis was very good. On Monday, we had an appointment with the neurologist who came highly recommended by my daughter who worked in the medical field. The neurologist was related to her boss, so we felt privileged and it appeared that his new medical team was coming together nicely. The neurologist prognosis was not good, the MRI detected a few dry spots of blood in his head which was indicative of previous strokes that we were unaware of. After having such a bad experience with the doctors and the hospital associated with the university, he was blessed with the best nurses, doctors and specialists in Maryland. We were blessed with a new and great team of doctors, and Rick had completely disassociated himself with the university and never went back to D.C. He was still insured by them, but he now went to a Maryland hospital and Maryland doctors. The Lord provided the hope and confidence we yearned for. Praise God!

Blessed is the man who trusts in the Lord, and whose hope is the Lord. Jeremiah 17:7

If there wasn't one thing, there was another. I was listening to the news and couldn't believe my ears, a plane crash, who, when, I was confused, picking up bits and pieces of the news forecast, but I eventually heard it all. Dr. Collison and his son were killed in his private plane piloted by Dr. Collison. Shortly after he died, Dr. Dixon, a doctor in his office suddenly passed away from a heart attack. Just like that, they were both gone, and we were devastated. Rick was especially hurt since he wanted Dr. Dixon to be his new primary care physician and Dr. Collison was his new heart doctor. He couldn't believe that he had lost two good doctors back to back that he truly liked. Our great team of doctors were falling apart just as fast as it came together and that was extremely discouraging. This had become our way of life, it was always something. We were right back where we started from. "Life is unpredictable," I said, "life is hard, but we are his children, we are right with God, and live under his protection so we're good, God will deliver us. By the grace of God, we'll find new and great doctors."

Many are the afflictions of the righteous, but the LORD delivers him out of them all. Psalm 34:19

While Rick and I spent a lot of time together we both enjoyed having our own places, yet my home had become ours. I will have to take this situation one day at a time and I could not make any promises or commitments, but I was going to try to take care of Rick if it did not interfere or conflict with my job. At the beginning and understandably so, Rick was stuck on the pity pot. I gave him a short pass since the doctors said that was normal. In the meantime, I was impatiently waiting for the antidepressants and antianxiety meds to kick in because I was ready to throw in the towel. I had zero tolerance for crybabies or people who pitied themselves. It was bad enough that I had no idea how to process all of this or how to proceed and on top of that he was acting like a five-year-old kid. I did not know how to take care of someone so sad and uncooperative. He was one miserable man and he was working on my reserve nerve. I was ready to walk out on him and I wanted absolutely no parts of this at all. I was not giving up, but I did not feel sorry for him either, and I never signed up for this to begin with. I did not understand his attitude when he was given a second chance at life. He was rebellious, negative and refused to take occupational and physical therapy. I couldn't help someone who didn't want to help himself. He really didn't want to be helped. Furthermore, I was not equipped to take care of someone as sick as he was, and he was way too angry, unappreciative, and discouraged. He was bringing me down with his bad attitude and negative energy. I had been running back and forth to the doctors since he was released from the hospital, so I am sleep deprived, exhausted, and I still had to go to work. He wasn't making this easy. I just couldn't do this. If he wanted my help then he needed to act like it and pull himself together, get some strength, faith, and hope from somewhere because I was losing patience, real fast, and if I couldn't do it, no one could. I had the patience of a saint, and zero tolerance for anyone who gives up. He had the wrong attitude for someone in his predicament and he needed to humble himself. "You had a stroke, you are not dead," I said, "God saved you so that you could get up and keep going. You were saved by the grace of God, and your life was spared. God is enabling you to get up. Praise God! When you are praising God, you won't be able to stay down. God enables you to get up when you think you can't.

Therefore humble yourselves under the mighty hand of God, that He may exalt you in due time, casting all your care upon Him, for He cares for you. 1 Peter 5:6-7

All the years Rick and I were together I thought I really knew him, but I didn't know him at all. There was help available, but he didn't want any help. Rather than be thankful that he was alive, he was angry. I could not relate to that.

God's promises are proven by His power. When God makes a promise, He'll come through for you. God created the world in seven days, parted the Red Sea, brought a mighty flood upon the earth, knocked down the walls of Jericho, sent fire from Heaven to consume Elijah's sacrifice, calmed the storm, wrote the Ten Commandments, He rose from the grave, and more, all which demonstrates His promises and His powers. God's promises are powerful enough to change our lives now and eternally.

19

If I could only convince Rick to believe in God's promises and power, what a happier man he would be. He fought against all treatments and complained about everything all the time and the bottom line, he was afraid of dying and he was a man of little faith. He used his stroke as an excuse for living to die and being on death watch. He was making himself sicker and his life miserable. Hopefully a shot of Job will give him just the faith-lift he needs because he was in an extremely gloomy place and he was a real hard nut to crack. I ended the night with a gentle kiss and whispered: 'This too shall pass, I love you.'"

If you would prepare your heart, and stretch out your hands toward Him; if iniquity were in your hand, and you put it far away, and would not let wickedness dwell in your tents; then surely you could lift up your face without spot; yes, you could be steadfast, and not fear; because you would forget your misery, and remember it as waters that have passed away, and your life would be brighter than noonday. Though you were dark, you would be like the morning. Job 11:13-17

He believed in God, but he did not believe in miracles which meant that he did not truly believe that God could do all He said He could do. So, he was among those who believe in a higher being, but it was obvious that he did not trust Him fully, but I had to make him understand that if God said He's going to do it, he's going to do it. "You fall short of healing and recovering because of your mindset, and you don't believe that God can do what he said he can do," I said, "He's a miracle worker, you must trust him, be indwelt with the power and the will of God as well as the will to live. Focus

20

on God to give you strength. If you trust Him, He will come through in every situation. Seek God for every need and direction you desire. He will intervene in your life and point you in the right direction, he will show you how to live your life to your very best. Whatever you're going through, He will bring you through it." Somehow, I had to penetrate that thick skull of his, but I also had to practice what I preached because we were totally losing control of our lives. Our lives changed overnight. Rick was losing his grip and fast. He was drowning in his own sorrow. He was depressed, miserable, bitter and angry. He was making me unhappy, so I did not want to even be around him. To him, it was easier to give up than it was to keep going. He did not feel he was giving up, he felt he was fighting a losing battle. He was blocking his blessings and healing. "Satan is the adversary in your ear," I said, "telling you that you will never get any better, but the Holy Spirit is in charge." There was little powering forward or reasoning with him. He considered his life to be over. All I could do was cry to God, "Please give me strength, give him strength, Oh Lord, and please give us strength. Help him, Lord to rise up and let him see the light at the end of the tunnel."

The Lord is my light and my salvation. Psalm 27:1

I pushed him as hard as I could for as long as I could and until I couldn't push him anymore, all along, wearing myself out. By the grace of God, over time, we roughed it out to the point where he could walk with a cane and drive which made him overly confident—he thought he was well enough to stop taking physical therapy that he started late, and he never took occupational therapy which is probably why I had to dress him. The doctors had already concluded that he may never walk or work again as it was, he was walking which meant that he had exceeded the doctor's expectations, so I was upset and disappointed that he would not power forward. I loved him, but I didn't like him anymore. He was full of excuses. In my opinion, Rick had to care about himself first before he could care about anyone else. I do not doubt that it was difficult, life was harder than it has ever been for me too, but that was the time to be strong, not take the easy way out or give up. Not taking occupational therapy at all and not taking physical therapy like he should have been was setting him up for failure. "Body in motion stays in motion, body in rest stays in rest." Shaking my head, I thought to myself, "He is setting himself up to die a slow death." I could just feel it. I honestly believed that Rick could be healed and if not, God would provide him with what he needed to get through it. Rick, on the other hand, was not a true believer and I could see that it was going to take a lot more convincing.

But He was wounded for our transgressions, He was bruised for our iniquities; the chastisement for our peace was upon Him, and by His stripes we are healed. Isaiah 53:5

Difficulties and challenges motivated me, not discouraged me. Rick was often down, and I couldn't totally blame him because he was in rough shape, he had everything in the world wrong with him, but the reality was he was still very much alive. He had no hope or faith. I had no idea what to do but I knew I had to exercise more patience and I had to come up with ways to motivate him, stimulate his mind, and stir up love and good heartedness among us.

And let us consider one another in order to stir up love and good works. Hebrews 10:24

No one knows how they're going to react in a "life or death" situation until it happens to them. I was kind of feeling his blues, but I just couldn't share that moment with him because it would not have been healthy for him to have a crying partner. Rick cried enough on his own and he has reason to cry, but not to give up. He probably thought that I was insensitive, or had a bad bladder because I hide my tears and spent a lot of time in the bathroom and shower. He had no idea what I was going through. I told him: "God is giving you more time to get it right, and to get rid of your fears, God counts and bottles your tears so it's okay to cry. Pray to God, He can change your mind and have you thinking less about dying and more about living; less about being ill and more about healing. If you trust God, He could turn this thing around."

Salvation [belongeth] unto the LORD; thy blessing [is] upon thy people. Selah. Psalm 3:8

I had no idea how I would get through this, working and taking care of a sick man was way more than I could handle alone. Thank God for my daughter Dana who was skilled in lifting and pulling patients up and down the steps which is exactly what she did the day my niece, daughter and I had to take Rick for a MRI and he had to take Lorazepam to get through it. Well, he made it through the MRI fine but when we left he was lethargic and could hardly sit up in the wheelchair, instead he was sliding out of it and he couldn't hold his head up either. With his legs stretched straight out, we had to wrestle with transferring his dead weight from the

23

wheelchair to the car seat, buckle him in, get him out of the car, and up the stairs into the house where there were even more stairs. I would have fallen on my face if I had tried to pull him up all those steps like she did. She was a strong tiny something too, and I do not know what I would have done without her because I was useless when it came to Rick and stairs. Bless her heart. I had to undress, bathe and get him ready for bed after everyone left and that was a bit much for me. I prayed like I had never prayed before. I didn't even know I knew how to pray like that, but I needed all the help and prayer I could get.

For I, the LORD your God, will hold your right hand, saying to you, 'Fear not, I will help you.' Isaiah 41:13

Somehow, I had to learn how to balance work and home. I just had no idea how I was going to do it. I wasn't eating or sleeping and I was exhausted all the time. Time was of the essence, I needed to figure it out, with the quickness, because I had to go back to work the next day, Tuesday. It was hard accepting this new lifestyle. We went from being a vibrant youngish middle-aged couple who was traveling, loving and living life to the fullest to living a life of medicine, doctor appointments, fear, being afraid of another stroke, blood transfusions, congested heart failure, death, depression, anxiety, organ failure – living like an elderly couple and forced to take it one day at a time. No matter what, I was frustrated and discouraged and I knew I couldn't be. I sure wished money grew on trees, so I could hire someone. God was the only one I had, so He was the only one that could help me.

And the LORD, He is the One who goes before you. He will be with you, He will not leave you nor forsake you; do not fear nor be dismayed. Deuteronomy 31:8

I never planned on Rick getting sick or imagined me being his caregiver, not this soon because he did have some bad eating habits that I commented on several times, but they went upon death ears because he still ate shrimp foo young almost every day for lunch and the remainder as a dinner appetizer before dinner, literally every day for months, until he couldn't walk due to too much iodine, but the soy sauce raises blood pressure, and rice was too much carbs plus he ordered extra shrimp. Why should I have to suffer, I didn't do anything wrong and I was in the prime of my life. I didn't like lawyers but I loved my job. I loved working, getting out of the house, having my own money, being independent, and I wasn't ready to stop working. I began to make excuses. Perhaps I should've taken a break after Nick or maybe this was karma because of the way I dumped him, but he should've left when he had the chance rather than being a freeloader. I began to feel a pattern with just dumping people though and I was feeling bad about it this time. I prayed on it, but still concluded that Rick had to go because I was not quitting my job. My house had way too many steps, his house had way less steps, but it was way too far for me to commute plus his stepdaughter, her husband and kids were living there now. Rick talked about putting his stepdaughter and her family out, but I said, "hell no, I am a no drama mama and if you put her out, you'll be home alone, and you need help. Orange is just too far in the boonies for me." All Rick wanted was me, but I couldn't do it. I loved him dearly, probably more now being sick than when he was well, but I couldn't wrap my head around all of this, it was just too serious, too much, and too soon. I knew that love never gives up, losses faith, and endures through every circumstance but I wasn't feeling his whole caregiving thing.

Love suffers long and is kind; love does not envy; love does not parade itself, is not puffed up; does not behave rudely, does not seek its own, is not provoked, thinks no evil; does not rejoice in iniquity, but rejoices in the truth; bears all things, believes all things, hopes all things, endures all things. 1 Corinthians 13:7

I wasn't feeling it. In the meantime, Rick was feeling defeated, defenseless, and in a very dark place. Financially, he was struggling and needing money until his disability was approved. He was basically forced to give up his D.C. apartment because he could no longer afford it, plus it was a waste of money anyway since he was at my house all the time. Rick felt as though giving up his apartment was a form of failure, and he could not figure out why he had a stroke, and now he was faced with losing his apartment. He felt as though his whole world was falling apart. All I could say was, "Life can change in an instant, sometimes life sucks, and bad things happen to good people. It's all a part of life." It was time he received a blesson about money and possessions, straight out of the bible:

"Don't store up treasures here on earth, where moths eat them and rust destroys them, and where thieves break in and steal. Store your treasures in heaven, where moths and rust cannot destroy, and thieves do not break in and steal. Wherever your treasure is, there the desires of your heart will also be. "Your eye is like a lamp that provides light for your body. When your eye is healthy, your whole body is filled with light. But when your eye is unhealthy, your whole

body is filled with darkness. And if the light you think you have is actually darkness, how deep that darkness is! "No one can serve two masters. For you will hate one and love the other; you will be devoted to one and despise the other. You cannot serve God and be enslaved to money. "That is why I tell you not to worry about everyday life—whether you have enough food and drink, or enough clothes to wear. Isn't life more than food, and your body more than clothing? Look at the birds. They don't plant or harvest or store food in barns, for your heavenly Father feeds them. And aren't you far more valuable to him than they are? Can all your worries add a single moment to your life? "And why worry about your clothing? Look at the lilies of the field and how they grow. They don't work or make their clothing, yet Solomon in all his glory was not dressed as beautifully as they are. And if God cares so wonderfully for wildflowers that are here today and thrown into the fire tomorrow, he will certainly care for you. Why do you have so little faith? "So don't worry about these things, saying, 'What will we eat? What will we drink? What will we wear?' These things dominate the thoughts of unbelievers, but your heavenly Father already knows all your needs. Seek the Kingdom of God above all else, and live righteously, and he will give you everything you need. "So don't worry about tomorrow, for tomorrow will bring its own worries. Today's trouble is enough for today." Matthew 6:19-34.

"That is exactly why we are not supposed to get attached to material things," I said, "things that we can lose so don't be disappointed about losing stuff because what goes down can come back up. Right now, you just need to roll with the punches, and trust in God. Your life has done a 360-degree turn. You can always get another apartment if you need one later, you really don't need one right now, but one day when you are healthier and can afford it, and you can live on your own and alone, then it shall be, but in the meantime, it is, what it is, and you must be practical and spend wisely. You have enough on your plate; you do not need anything extra to worry about, especially additional expenses. What you need is not for sell, it's priceless – you cannot buy health, love, peace, joy, happiness, or eternal life. Keep your primary focus on Jesus, your health, your overall well-being."

And this is the testimony: that God has given us eternal life, and this life is in His Son. He who has the Son has life; he who does not have the Son of God does not have life. These things I have written to you who believe in the name of the Son of God, that you may know that you have eternal life, and that you may continue to believe in the name of the Son of God. 1 John 5:11-13

I was all Rick had so all by my lonesome, I packed up his apartment. It was in the city, close to the subway, work, downtown, restaurants and shops. Now, I could really see why he was sick. His kitchen cabinets and refrigerator were stocked with all the wrong things–sugary cereals, canned goods, processed foods, chips, candy and meats. After I finished packing his apartment, I organized a moving crew to move his belongings from the apartment to a storage unit in Virginia. My plate was full, about to run over.

God is our refuge and strength, a very present help in trouble. Psalm 46:1

Moving forward, every day was unpredictable, so I was never able to figure out what my day was going to be like. Working, taking care of Rick, organizing meals for him to eat while I was at work, and trying to stay on top of everything that I had to do, I was totally burnt out. I was only one person. Rick had become my priority and it appeared that I was stuck with taking care of him whether I wanted to or not. Although I had made up my mind that he had to go, I also had to get him situated to go. I couldn't just throw him out, it just wasn't that easy. Reluctantly, he finally decided to agree to disagree, and go live with one of his three children with the hopes that at least one or all of them would pitch in and take turns caring for him like my family had done when my mother could no longer live alone. It is what families do. I couldn't understand why I should turn my life upside down or quit my job, I was not prepared to make such a huge, life-altering commitment, I just couldn't do it, and I wasn't going to do it. I had an attitude— let his children make some sacrifices.

When parent-children roles are reversed, children should see their sick parent as a blessing, not a burden.

This is one time that I was glad that I was the girlfriend and not the wife but nonetheless it really bothered me to say no. Even Rick often said that I needed to learn to say "no" sometimes. I said, "no," and I meant it this time. He needed way more than I could give him. I could not afford to quit my job. All I could do was pray for strength, healing and more family support but this was not the time to be weak.

Therefore I take pleasure in infirmities [illness], in reproaches [criticism], in needs [necessities], in persecutions [harassment], in distresses [pain], for Christ's sake. For when I am weak, then I am strong. 2 Corinthians 12:10

When you have children, they should step up to the plate and pull their weight especially if they are all their parents have. They took care of them, why shouldn't they look out for their parents? Unfortunately, we do not ask that these roles be reversed, it just happens and when it does we will never be prepared. Therefore, we must pray and get ready to do what our parents would expect us to do or would do for us if the shoe was on the other foot. It's another challenge, it's another test and it's all a part of life.

Knowing that the testing of your faith produces patience. James 1:3

Rick was feeling afflicted, rejected, unwanted and that was painful for me to watch. I did not want to complicate his life any more than it already was, but it wasn't that his kids couldn't do it, they didn't want to do it and they refused to do it. Well, I didn't want to do it either. I was already crying in the shower as it was to avoid him seeing me emotionally distressed. Also, I did not want him to feel lonely, abandoned or rejected, but I was feeling overwhelmed, so I was trying hard to stay out of my feelings.

Being alone and lonely are two different things. One can be home alone but not lonely, and one can even feel lonely in a large crowd. Loneliness is an emotion caused by feeling separated from another person or persons and the sense of separation is severely felt by those suffering with loneliness.

I did not want Rick to slip into a deeper sadness or depression. I did not want him to be sick and feeling alone like he was or feeling as though he was without a friend in the world, no one cared or was the least bit concerned about whether he was dead or alive. I loved him dearly and I prayed that he would find peace.

Elect according to the foreknowledge of God the Father, through sanctification of the Spirit, unto obedience and sprinkling of the blood of Jesus Christ: Grace unto you, and peace, be multiplied. 1 Peter 1:2

At the same time, I had to protect me. This was my life and if I gave up my life for Rick at this juncture I would totally resent him and the whole caregiving process in the long run, things would not have gone smoothly, or have a good outcome because I just was not on board or ready and I was not sure I ever would be. It was a lot to ask of someone and it was a lot for me to think about. I would continue to seek answers through prayer. It may sound selfish, but I did not want to put myself in a situation that I would regret later. I refused to set myself up to be miserable, and I was not going to do anything that I did not want to do. Let his children do their part and if they fail I will revisit the subject again at that time. In the interim his children needed to take heed to their biblical responsibility and honor their father.

"Honor your father and mother," which is the first commandment with promise: "that it may be well with you and you may live long on the earth." Ephesians 6:2-3

His children would undoubtedly honor their mother, so I was prayerful and hopeful that they would extend the same olive branch to their father. Rick was a giver and his children should have been more supportive and nicer to him. He said they didn't want to be bothered with him, they were just going through the motions. I felt horrible for him, but he and his kids just needed more time and I needed to mind my business.   He and his kids needed to work on their relationship.

Bear with each other and forgive if any of you has a grievance against someone.   Forgive as the Lord forgave you. Colossians 3:13

Chapter 2

Living-to-Die

I couldn't take Rick's living-to-die attitude. I was not kicking him to the curb like he thought, no way, no how, that just wasn't me, and my heart wouldn't let me. He agreed to disagree and go live with his kids, so I put the plan in motion and packed his belongings. To me, we were taking a break, but to him, it was a break-up. He was all in his feelings, and I was not surprised. He took everything to the extreme and negatively. He felt that I didn't want him and once I got him out of my house I would be rid of him forever. It was sad, and I felt bad for him, but I could not change his mind for him or predict the future, and I was truly hopeful that he would have a breakthrough and want to live instead of dying and being on death watch. He had my head spinning and my heart was heavy.

Turn Yourself to me, and have mercy on me, for I am desolate and afflicted. The troubles of my heart have enlarged; bring me out of my distresses! Psalm 25:16-17

I couldn't tell him anything. To him, it was dooms day, the end. He was not going to be out of my life, but I couldn't change his thoughts. I knew he would never be whole again and he would be more independent and much better off without me. I spoiled him rotten and he was too dependent on me for everything after the stroke and he really needed to work on himself and at least work on regaining some independence and mobility. I was sure that he had made the right decision for now and he would fully accept it and merely adjust to it, eventually. He was able to drive, move around with his walker or cane. He required some assistance with meal preparation because he couldn't stand for long periods of time, the right-side weakness was no longer affecting his equilibrium, so he had more control over his balance and the nerves in his hand was still a work-in-progress. One good thing, he was not falling anymore.

Come close to God, and God will come close to you. Wash your hands, you sinners; purify your hearts, for your loyalty is divided between God and the world. Let there be tears for what you have done. Let there be sorrow and deep grief. Let there be sadness instead of laughter, and gloom instead of joy. Humble yourselves before the Lord, and he will lift you up in honor. James 4:8-10

Overall, he was doing better than he was when he first came home. Progress was slow, but progress, nonetheless. It appeared he was on his way to making a good recovery, and he still needed to be careful to prevent having another stroke, or adding a heart attack to his growing list of illnesses. He did not need anything new or anymore setbacks. Whether he and I were together or not, I will still be there for him. Rick acts like a victim, and he is not, he is a stroke survivor, a victor. I couldn't work and take care of him because he could not be left home alone plus I couldn't call out anymore because I had no more leave. I could not afford to take leave without pay or jeopardize being fired. His stroke had already taken us by surprise and threw us for a loop, so I couldn't imagine another one. I was truly afraid of him having another stroke, a heart attack or dying, while under my watch, so moving was not his choice, he had to go. He being sick was making me sick and I could not afford to be sick right now. Rick was on disability with his job, and it would be at least two years before his social security disability would begin, so I refused to give up my security and independence, but somehow, I still had to work it all out. Moving him away was just a temporary solution, we needed a resolution. I was praying without ceasing that God turns his health around, so that everything did not fall on me.

God's thoughts are higher than the world's thoughts and his ways are higher than our ways. He is a way-maker. Only He can make a way out of no way.

I was beginning to sound like a broken record but who was going to take care of me while I was taking care of him? Who was going to be the caregiver's caregiver? The reality was if he weren't with "his kids" then it would be all on me. All I wanted was for his children to at least try, that's all, just try. It was three of them, it was only one of me and it was just way too much for me and just like his kids, my kids had families, responsibilities, jobs and lives too. I tried it and it did not work for me. The same two kids who picked him up from the hospital (when he was released after the stroke) arrived at my home to pick him up to take him to Virginia. Before leaving, he gave me a kiss and whispered in my ear, "I don't want to go, I love you, and you know I don't want to live with my kids. Why are you making me do this?" I thought we were passed this, so he obviously did not really take me seriously. He agreed to disagree, and it was time to go. We had already talked about it, I had made myself perfectly clear and I was not talking about it anymore. I knew he didn't want to go, but he had no choice. All his

35

children lived in the same area or close enough to each other to help their dad. He was hopeful that his children would be more caring, helpful, loving, supportive and respectful because he felt he had done his best as a father and raised his children well, and now he was feeling alone and really needed them. He merely wanted them to treat him the way he treats them, with nothing but love and kindheartedness. He would never mistreat them in anyway. There was nothing he wouldn't do for either of his children.

And you, fathers, do not provoke your children to wrath, but bring them up in the training and admonition of the Lord. Ephesians 6:4

Rick was the most loveable and chilled guy I ever met, and he deserved better from his children. Just as expected, he wasn't happy about his new living arrangement, not at all. As a matter of fact, he was miserable. From day one he complained and there was nothing that I could do about it. He needed to call a family meeting and tell his children his needs and expectations, not me. He hated living with his stepdaughter so much he tried putting another double-wide trailer on his property, but the zoning commissioner denied his application. He said he felt like an outcast with his family and unwanted by his daughter and her family, as though he was imposing on them, so he was contemplating moving in with his son who was single, no kids, he had an extra room, and he was self-employed therefore seldom home so Rick would have more privacy. I know he was craving his solitude. At least he was exploring other options rather than expecting to return to my house. He was trying and that's all I could ask of him. I was prayerful and hopeful that his children would be happy that their father was still alive and I prayed that they would be more proactive and hands-on. Whether they realized it or not, their father desperately needed them, he was hurting, frail, he could have died, and he still wasn't totally out of the woods.

You shall always be children in the eyes of your parents and in the eyes of the Lord. Honoring your parents may be a way to measure your honor, obedience and faithfulness.

After a few weeks, he moved in with his son. That was a good thing. I still felt strongly that it was good for him to be around his family and children, so I was happy for him. Rick was such a good guy he would much rather find housing than inconvenience his stepdaughter and her family. I was on the outside looking in, so I was shaking my head because even as a very sick man he was thinking of others. It was equally as obvious who his stepdaughter was thinking about. I just couldn't figure out why he was trying to find a place to live when he already had a place to live. Common courtesy and love for her father should have moved his stepdaughter and her family out, but it didn't. Personally, I felt his meekness was being mistaken for weakness. I prayed that God would comfort him, protect him from evil, and make things right in his life.

May the Lord bless you and protect you. May the Lord smile on you and be gracious to you. May the Lord show you his favor and give you his peace, the LORD bless you and keep you; the LORD make His face shine upon you and be gracious to you; the LORD lift up His countenance upon you, and give you peace. Numbers 6:24-26

He was out of my house but not out of my life. He was only a phone call away, so we spoke on the phone daily, sometimes several times a day. He would mostly call to complain or to let me know where he was going. He was adamant about not living with his son for too long. He just didn't have much of a choice right now. However, according to Rick his son disliked and disowned him and claimed some other man as his father although he knew Rick was his biological father, so they had some deep underlying, and unresolved issues that only they could resolve and maybe this was as good a time as any to make amends. We must forgive to be forgiven.

For if you forgive men their trespasses, your heavenly Father will also forgive you. But if you do not forgive men their trespasses, neither will your Father forgive your trespasses. Matthew 6:14-15

Rick said that they have always had a rocky relationship, so I hoped that they would work out their differences before it was too late. Regardless of all the cons and complaints he was still there, and he was adjusting, surviving, being mobile, and showing signs of improvements. Nothing could stop him from being lonely and bored out of his wits, but he was doing better with his son than he did with his stepdaughter. He was complaining less about his son, probably because he was never home, and less people were around. He reiterated with every conversation that he did not want to live with any of his children because they did not want to be bothered with him and he couldn't blame them. Rick said, "It's unfair to expect my children to take care of a sick parent." I replied, "If it were their mother, they would do it, and if your son didn't want you there you wouldn't be there." "I'm homeless and homesick," he cried, "no one wants to be bothered with me, including you. I want to be with you, I want to come home, so I'm never going to be happy anywhere else. I'll never get well without you." That crushed me, but I couldn't allow him to put me on a guilt trip. It hadn't been that long, and he just needed more time. I said, "You better make the best of it because it isn't fair to me either."

Family and friends may disappoint or fail you, and enemies may even attack you, but God will be there until the very end to keep you lifted, so keep the faith, and never give up.

I knew he missed me, his maid, nurse, chef, companion, hugger, listener, life coach, spiritual advisor, counselor, caregiver, lover and best friend. Who wouldn't miss all that especially compared to what he was getting now? He wasn't even getting the time of day from his children. I explained to him repeatedly that I must work, and he could not be left home alone. Of course, he swore up and down that he could, but I wasn't taking any chances. There were so many things to consider and Rick was not capable of making any decisions on his own. I had way too many steps, I would have to get up extra early to prepare his meals, and get him situated upstairs for the day and it would interrupt my flow of getting myself ready for work every day and God forbid if there is a fire or emergency where he has to leave the house, he would not be able to get downstairs without assistance. That thought terrified me even more. I couldn't take a chance on him hurting himself. I think he found more complaints with both of his kids than he would have found in a nursing home, but he had more complaints while with his stepdaughter than son and probably because he did not have any children around at his son's house. Don't get me wrong, he loved his grandchildren immensely, but he wasn't himself and only wanted to be bothered when he wanted to be bothered. He also did not want his grandchildren to see or remember him as a sickly grandfather. It would have been much easier to put him in a home, however he made it clear, from the start that he was not going into a nursing home and he meant that. At this point, I was just like his kids, merely going through the motions. I cannot speak for his kids, but I was waiting on the Lord for direction. After all, He knew my load and what I was capable of handling.

Cast your burden on the LORD, and He shall sustain you; He shall never permit the righteous to be moved. Psalm 55:22

I remained optimistic but in Rick's eyesight, things weren't going to change. I believed that time heals everything, so I'll give them a little more time to work the kinks out. Rick deserved better. By the grace of God he was surviving without anyone's help. The highlight of his day was taking night drives to Walmart. He would call me, talk to me on the way there, while shopping, and on his ride back home. For him to be getting out was a plus and I was happy for him but sometimes, I spent so much time on the phone with him he might as well have still been living with me. I asked God to wrap his arms around him, keep him strong, healthy, and protected from evil and further sickness.

Have I not commanded you? Be strong and of good courage; do not be afraid, nor be dismayed, for the LORD your God is with you wherever you go. Joshua 1:9

I was livid when he eventually admitted to me that he was, eating carryout and fast food. Obviously, not following his diet like he should. His diet was a matter of life and death and he should be preparing his own meals. I was very disappointed that he was not taking his health or stroke more seriously and if he and his children didn't care, why the heck should I? I love him but that just gave me an excuse to take a real break from him, the stress and drama was just too much for me. I had to put it in the hands of the Lord. Rick was a distraction. There was nothing that I could do but continue to pray for him because he or his children obviously didn't care as much as I did. Rick didn't seem to have any intentions on doing the right thing where his health was concerned, and that is why he had a stroke in the first place, yet he had the audacity to be mad at God, bitter and angry because he had a stroke. It was his health and his life. I'm tired, all I could do was cry and pray, "Lord, heal his body, restore his health and renew his spirit, wrap him in your loving arms." The Lord nurses the sick and restores their health.

The LORD will strengthen him on his bed of illness; You will sustain him on his sickbed. Psalm 41:3

It was hard to ignore Rick, but it was the same old same old. He kept telling me I was all he had, and he continued to complain about his children not doing anything for him. I was tired of hearing it. I was not going to allow Rick to put any pressure on me before his children put forth any effort.

My little children, let us not love in word, neither in tongue; but in deed and in truth. 1 John 3:18

41

Nothing had changed on my end, he still needed assistance and I still had to work. His children still weren't stepping up to the plate. I wanted him to put his foot down but when I asked him why his children weren't working together to do more for him he only defended them as usual. "They have their own lives, their own families, responsibilities," he said, "and jobs, they just don't have time for me." I replied, "Your son is self-employed, single, no children so there is no excuse, he needs to make time. What about me? I have a family and job too. If I can make sacrifices, so can they." He did not have any expectations of his kids. That was frustrating, but nothing new because he was famous for making excuses for his children. He said, "They don't have the type of heart that you have nor the know-how, advocacy, patience, caregiving nature, medical knowledge or godliness to take care of a person as sick as me. They just don't know what to do or how to do it." "Neither did I," I responded, "at first, but I learned, and they can learn too if they wanted to. Stop making excuses for them, your youngest child works in a nursing home so stop making excuse for all of them. Keep the faith, baby because you don't have anyone on your side but Jesus and me."

Train up a child in the way he should go, and when he is old he will not depart from it. Proverbs 22:6

"They are your children," I continued, "and they need to at least put forth some effort, that is all I'm asking, just try before you quit. It is obvious that your children do not want to do it, but it's not that they can't do it, they just won't do it, and refuse to do it." He said he was lonely, he missed me and that his children could not fill that void or my shoes. I did not expect them to fill my shoes or any void and I felt bad that he did not have the family love and support that he needed, but neither did I. I had his and my bills to pay. I was home alone but I wasn't lonely. All I could do was shake my head and try not to get into my feelings, but it wasn't easy. I kept thinking about Rick needing my help. There was never any doubt that no one could take care of him like me because no one loved him like me, but the problem was I did not want to do it and I had made up my mind that I wasn't going to do it until I was ready to, if ever. I never say never because I never know and never is in the future, I can't predict the future, and I had not totally dismissed the caregiving idea. There was the possibility that I would change my mind or God would touch my heart in the future. I still felt horrible but not bad enough to commit to caregiving. As I walked through the park on my lunch hour, I prayed.

So He Himself often withdrew into the wilderness and prayed. Luke 5:16

As I prayed, I couldn't help but to think how I am always talking about somebody stepping up to the plate and here I was, not stepping up to the plate, so I was feeling somewhat guilty. As I walked I thought to myself, "Was it really my plate to step up to?" I answered myself too, "No, I am not married to him, so he is not my responsibility. I love him to life, but I need my job for real, I just can't quit my job like that, it would be crazy for me to do that." I'll continue to pray and ask for God's guidance.

Therefore, as the elect of God, holy and beloved, put on tender mercies, kindness, humility, meekness, long-

suffering; bearing with one another, and forgiving one another, if anyone has a complaint against another; even as Christ forgave you, so you also must do. But above all these things put on love, which is the bond of perfection. 1 Colossians 3:12-14

My feelings were getting the best of me. The word "love," kept surfacing. I had love on the brain. I questioned myself, "What's love got to do with it?" Since I had no one else to talk to, I talked and thought to myself a lot. I was thinking to myself, "Love is what binds us all together in perfect harmony. To become a fulltime caregiver meant that I would have to give up my entire life. I helped everybody, but I couldn't save the world. Rick had not been gone that long, and he was determined to be with me. I missed him because we were like two peas in a pod, we did everything together, he kept me real busy, and I will never forget, he gave me everything my heart desired, and I wish I could do the same for him. I began to question my loyalty and love for him. No doubt about it, Rick was a blessing, I loved and appreciated him with all my heart, but I just couldn't do what he was asking of me.

Delight yourself also in the Lord, and He shall give you the desires of your heart. Psalm 37:4

Being the compassionate person that I am, I began feeling selfish and guilty, so I decided to extend Rick an olive branch; I started helping him with grocery shopping, preparing healthy meals and laundry. Sometimes I would let him stay overnight if he appeared too weak or sick to drive alone. I was afraid something could happen to him on the road and he might not be able to get to safety in time. I was still relying on the power of prayer. Prayer always gave me clarity and guided me in the right direction. I had to do some soul searching as well. I had to dig deep down inside my heart. He had been gone a little over a month and I really didn't want him back right now because I knew I couldn't work and take care of him too. I just couldn't do it. As much as I hated to admit it, he was a burden. I did not want this responsibility or commitment. I was not up for the challenge. I was also enjoying the overtime, not having to rush home to cook and not wearing myself out taking care of a sick man, and the extra money was definitely a big plus. With Rick, it was like I had two jobs, I would leave my day job and home would be my night job. No one should relate home to work. More than anything, I was not prepared to watch another loved one die, not just yet.

Grief is the price we pay for the love of a loved one; it is a necessary evil. Take time to grieve but you do not want it to become complicated grief which is an indication that you're unable to work through it alone and perhaps need professional help moving forward to the final stage, the healing process.

It hadn't been a year since my mom's death, so I was still grieving her passing. This whole situation with Rick was out of my control. I had no idea what the future might hold, and I was not about to put my life on hold for anybody. I decided to seriously take a real break. My conscience was saying don't let go, but let God do what He do.

Hear, my son, and receive my sayings, and the years of your life will be many. I have taught you in the way of wisdom; I have led you in right paths. When you walk, your steps will not be hindered, and when you run, you will not stumble. Take firm hold of instruction, do not let go. Proverbs 4:10

"If you have a bird and set it free, if it comes back, it was meant to be and if it doesn't, it was never yours to begin with" is one of my favorite quotes that came to mind. I was talked out and tired of repeating myself. Rick was not a happy camper but what else was new? At this point in his life everything irritated him. I really felt bad because he had stuck by me for years, encouraged me to write, provided me with a quiet environment for writing, purchased books and accompanied me wherever I needed to go to promote and market my books. He was my main supporter and biggest fan. Again, what he did for me, and what he was asking me to do was a horse of another color. Or was it? I was not obligated to him. He was asking me to give up my life and as much as he didn't want to be around his children, he had to admit that he might be better off with them than me in terms of his independence. He could also get to know them, and see them for who they really were. It wouldn't hurt to build a stronger bond with one another. I just wanted Rick to have an intimate relationship with God so that he could hear God's voice, bring things to pass, and get his life back – it starts with his children because he desperately needed their love and support, if nothing else.

Be anxious for nothing, but in everything by prayer and supplication, with thanksgiving, let your requests be made known to God. Philippians 4:6

Although Rick wasn't living with me he still needed me, and I was there for him, but I really didn't want to be needed or wanted the way he wanted and needed me. Be careful what you ask for. I had asked God to send me a good, faithful man that would really love, want, need, and adore me. I couldn't be mad at Rick because God gave me just what I asked for. Next time, I'll be way more specific. In the meantime, we'll just have to wait and see where God takes us from here. Of course, Rick is way better off in God's hands than anyone else's.

For our light affliction, which is but for a moment, is working for us a far more exceeding and eternal weight of glory, while we do not look at the things which are seen, but at the things which are not seen. For the things which are seen are temporary, but the things which are not seen are eternal. 2 Corinthians 4:17-18

I really didn't want to hear any complaints about his children, his health or otherwise. I just wanted some peace and quiet, some normalcy back into our lives. Rick was not the same person, so everything was different for his children too. He had lost his independence and he needed to talk to them about his expectations and needs. It may have seemed like a long time to him, but he hadn't been gone that long. No one was trying, he or his children. The stroke really did affect his brain, and what kind of kids did he born? They sure aren't family-oriented. As a matter of fact, they are quite cold. His thought patterns were the total opposite of the way he used to be. There wasn't anything that I could do about his situation now. I had no relationship with his children and I had to work. What did he want me to do? I was not a healer, I was not God and money did not grow on trees or fall out of the sky. I wasn't the one with the answers, he needed Jesus.

Because He has inclined His ear to me, therefore I shall call upon Him as long as I live. Psalm 116:2

Conversations with Rick would bring me down and make me feel awful so I wanted to avoid him at all cost but I couldn't because he would give up on himself but he wouldn't dare give up on me or our relationship. I did not pity him but provided him with faith-lifts throughout the day. I concluded that I had to stay out of my feelings and stand strong in my convictions. I just wasn't ready to be a caregiver or nurse, it was as simple as that, but I was genuinely concerned and honestly cared about his health and well-being. I still felt as though he was not my responsibility. No matter what, I felt guilty, it had me feeling down emotionally and I would cry about not being able to help him at this critical time in his life. I questioned myself day in and day out. Can I help him? Should I help him? Am I being selfish? Is this something God wants me to do? I didn't want to miss any 'Jesus Calling' opportunities. I even thought there was the possibility that I was pissed and/or angry at him for getting sick, and changing our lives as a reason why I didn't want to take care of him. I wasn't sure anymore what I felt except I loved him and wanted to help him stay encouraged and hopeful. Deep down inside, I knew I should be doing more but I was adamant about keeping my distance. Never judge others for their decisions or say what you would or would not do because you never know what you will do until you're confronted with the situation.

Judge not, that you be not judged. Matthew 7:1

When Rick became sick, I expected him to have more faith because before the stroke, he always appeared so strong and independent. I'm a caregiver by nature, so it wasn't so much the caregiving aspect of it as it was quitting my job, and giving up my life to watch Rick die. I would lose my independence, become dependent on Rick's disability income, and put limitations on the lifestyle I had become accustomed to. I saw no future in that at all. I really did not know what to do. God forbid, I were to get sick or miss out on my 'Jesus Calling'. God's message was clear, the greatest love is shown by giving the gift of life, whether it is caregiving, adoption, organ donation, or personal sacrifice.

Greater love hath no man than this, that a man lay down his life for his friends. John 15:13

I was trying not to be a hindrance to God. I did not want to hinder Him from showing us his will by being focused and preoccupied with doing things our way rather than God's way. God is our heavenly father. You would never expect your children to do the right thing if you never showed them what the right way was, would you? Same thing with God, how does He expect me to know something if He doesn't show me? He had a plan before He ever created me. If it is God's will, I will know sooner or later. I was anxious to know. I will be patient and wait on the Lord to reveal His will for me, to me.

For this reason we also, since the day we heard it, do not cease to pray for you, and to ask that you may be filled with the knowledge of His will in all wisdom and spiritual understanding. Colossians 1:9

A Very Long Goodbye

In trying to cope with Rick and his situation, I couldn't help but to draw strength from my dad's experience. He had an amputated leg and was blind in one eye but you would never have known it. We called him the bionic man and he was a great dancer too with one leg. In addition, he was a football coach for the Boys and Girls Club in DC. My dad's attitude was "I lost one leg, God gave me two, so I still got another one." Unfortunately, he died at 51 but he had a very positive attitude even as a young dying man. Rick had to surrender his fears. He had a lot to be thankful for, he had all his limbs. My father taught me that God did not give us a spirit of fear. "Fear blocks your ability to think clearly," he said, "it is a brain crusher and a mind killer."

For God has not given us a spirit of fear, but of power and of love and of a sound mind. 2 Timothy 1:7

Rick was a creature of habit but sometimes he was also full of surprises. I was deeply touched when I received flowers at work and a very sweet message that read: "Missing and thinking of you, always and forever, Rick," of course. When he called to confirm that I had received his flowers, he said he wanted to marry me and was seriously looking for a place for us to live. I laughed and told him that the telephone was not the place to propose. He laughed and said, "You were the one who said I needed to be more spontaneously so roll with me baby, and give me a break, will you marry me? Nothing is normal about us anyway. I can't get on my knees, I'm in a wheelchair, remember?" We both laughed, we said our "I love you" to each other, I thanked him for the flowers and told him how beautiful they were, and hung up the phone. Rick was looking and feeling pretty good these days and in very good spirits, so I didn't want to bust his bubble. I was happy because at one point he had drained me so bad I felt as though I needed a support group. He was totally ignoring the fact that we were no longer together. I did not want to talk to him every day, three or four times a day and see him two three or four times a week. I really wanted to help him, and I probably was giving him mixed signals.

The ultimate lesson all of us have to learn is unconditional love, which includes not only others but ourselves as well. Dr. Elisabeth Kubler-Ross

Our love used to be magical. Nothing was complicated. I was happy that he was doing something as opposed to being on death watch and waiting to die, but he was too overwhelming and needy. I was moving forward, not backwards. Regardless to Rick spoiling me and giving me all my hearts desires when he was able to, I still did not feel I owed him anything. I knew God was working behind the scenes, so I prayed without ceasing that God would continue to restore his health and renew his spirit.

When the sun was setting, all those who had any that were sick with various diseases brought them to Him; and He laid His hands on every one of them and healed them. And demons also came out of many, crying out and saying, "You are the Christ, the Son of God!" Luke 4:40-41

No matter what your needs are or what you're going through God will deliver you! It's our choice to receive it. One thing, Rick was determined to get his own place. He withdrew the necessary funds from his retirement, found an apartment and moved in, with the quickness. I was thrilled with his new attitude and energy level and I was hopeful for his recovery. The deluxe one-bedroom apartment was a straight shot to my job (in DC at the Watergate). That was the old Rick that I was used to, a real go-getter, and always making things happen. He was doing much better than I could ever imagine. For him to go out and find a place so quickly was remarkable and progress on a huge scale. I was proud to see him regain some independence and making such progress on his own. That was a bold move for Rick.

"For I know the plans that I have for you," declares the LORD, "plans for welfare and not for calamity to give you a future and a hope." Jeremiah 29:11

The following weekend I made a date to spend the entire weekend with him. He was ecstatic. I packed my bag the night before and took it to work with me. He was waiting outside my job when I got off from work, just like old times. We stopped at the grocery store, got our food, my wine and headed to his place. The apartment was in a great complex that housed mostly marines stationed at Quantico. Although I genuinely felt as though the storm had turned into a beautiful rainbow, I still wasn't ready to give up my house and my job and I did not want to be pressured or even discuss it. I also did not want to be torn between two homes, his and mine. Also, I did not want him to get it twisted–I was an encourager, not an enabler. He better recognizes, God was his enabler. "Help me, guide me, Lord because I'm in between a rock and a hard place trying to guide Rick. I put him in Your hands, Lord," I prayed.

Commit everything you do to the Lord. Trust him, and he will help you. Psalm 37:5

I had worked hard to save Rick's kidneys but eventually the nephrologist's prognosis wasn't good. He was diagnosed with end stage renal disease and it was time for him to start dialysis, something we had dreaded for years. Of course, he didn't want to take dialysis, who would, but he did not have a choice anymore. He would rather have his kidneys fail than start dialysis which meant he would rather die than take dialysis. I advised him to ask God, "What is his plan and will for you? Ask God to give you wisdom to deal with what you're going through. I cannot explain why bad things happen to good people, it just does. Perhaps in our situation, God wanted to change your direction—our direction. God has a plan for our lives and when we deviate from our predestined steps, or make decisions without God, we are expressing personal pride and behaving as though we do not need Him. What I do know is that the Holy Spirit is there to give us direction and provision, and we have the will of God, so it's okay to ask Him to make decisions in your life and express his will for your life. He is interested in you looking your best, feeling your best, being your best and doing your best because you represent the son of God so every aspect of your life matters to Him. If we do not choose God's direction we choose a lesser direction. Sometimes God has worked out something on our behalf that we don't even know about, and He's waiting on us to come to Him because He already knows everything about us and while we are trying to figure it out, He has already worked it out. I don't have all the answers, I can't predict the future, and I sure can't read the mind of the Holy Spirit, but what I can do is allow God to express his love to us and move in our lives.

When times are good, be happy; but when times are bad, consider this: God has made the one as well as the other. Therefore, no one can discover anything about their future. Ecclesiastes 7:14

God allows adversity to get our attention, adversity reminds us of our weaknesses, God knows how to weaken us, not to keep us weak, but so that we will be reminded of our strengths, and that sin has its penalties. God is dependable, trustworthy and always there especially in your greatest needs. Moving forward, face life knowing that God is in this with you and He will walk with you every step of the way, every day to get you through it. Reading the bible can help strengthen you in your loving relationship to the almighty God and Jesus and there is a load limit. He knows what you can and cannot take and he will not put any more on you than you can bear. That's a promise. It can be an opportunity, or it can be an obstacle." He looked bewildered and asked, "How do you know so much about God?" I answered, "God gets us ready to serve him in different ways. If we have been comforted by God, we have the ability to comfort others." "Really," he asked. "Yes," I replied, "really, simply by serving the Lord and being comforted by the Lord gives you the ability to help and comfort others." "Wow," he said, "You are an earth angel, so sweet and patient." I replied, "Everything happens for a reason and I think God is working on my patience. I may not be perfect, but my attitude and actions will always reflect my godliness. God's people are blessed to bless others."

Praise be to the God and Father of our Lord Jesus Christ,
the Father of compassion and the God of all comfort, who
comforts us in all our troubles, so that we can comfort
those in any trouble with the comfort we ourselves receive
from God. 2 Corinthians 1:3-4

I grew up in the church, I had to go, and we had no choice.
If we did not go to church, we could not go outside, to the
movies or anywhere else. Even if we visited my aunt, my
grandmother and great grandmother, I still had to go to
Sunday school and church every Sunday, no excuses. When
it comes to God, no excuses from you because God will
make your disability, give you credibility." He grinned and
said, "You always know what to say to make me smile and
feel better. Thank you." I replied, "Anytime! Just
remember God answers prayers, so pray without ceasing.
He also puts words in my mouth and that's how I always
know what to say."

Creating the praise of the lips. Peace, peace to him who is
far and to him who is near," Says the LORD, "and I will
heal him." Isaiah 57:19

I wanted Rick to see that even if he were to die, God forbid,
he needed to trust God if he wanted to live in peace as well
as to die in peace rather than be in the type of turmoil he was
experiencing. We had done so well for so long. For at least
two and a half years we were able to keep dialysis at bay.
After too many congested heart failure episodes to count,
and 44 blood transfusions, we knew it was inevitable, so here
we are. Praise God for answering that prayer, it's been a
very long time coming, but He's always on time. That
confirmation from the Holy Spirit energized me and gave me

the faith to stay strong. God chooses what's best, the right time, and the right way.

In the day when I cried out, You answered me, and made me bold with strength in my soul. Psalm 138:3

Rick went to his dialysis treatments kicking and screaming, all the way. He hated it. Half the day would be gone unless we went very early, so we spent a lot of 5:00 a.m. Saturday mornings at dialysis and I would wait for him in the lobby for four hours because whenever I left he gave everyone a hard time. He could be a pain in the behind when he wanted to be.

Fear not, for I am with you; be not dismayed, for I am your God. I will strengthen you, yes, I will help you, and I will uphold you with My righteous right hand. Isaiah 41:10

Hemodialysis was very hard on Rick. After dialysis treatment, he was zapped of all his fluid and energy. It would leave him lying around and not feeling well so I decided to stay over until Monday morning and commute from his place and return there that evening just to make sure he was okay and could be left alone before I returned to my home for the week. He was really looking swollen and uncomfortable, but he refused to go to the hospital. He was tired of going to the hospital because every time he went, he was admitted. When I stayed at his place, I had two options, I could slug for free riding as an additional passenger, so the driver could ride the HOV lane or I could take the commuter bus which coincidentally and literally went from Rick's apartment to my job for $22 a day roundtrip. The commute wasn't that bad and ironically my boss paid for my transportation to and from work, it was just cheaper to commute from Maryland to DC than from Virginia to DC, so I would miss the surplus cash from my employee transportation benefit. In any event, it was a blessing and I was thankful I had it to spare and share.

Happiness is only real when shared. Christopher McCandless

I began to visit Rick regularly, every weekend and I remained adamant about not moving there because the traffic was horrendous, and I never wanted to live in Virginia anyway since residents are required to pay real estate and personal property taxes. Also, I wasn't on board with quitting my job yet. Although the commute did give me some quiet time to myself and I could write in peace. I continued praying for God to shine His light on my path.

You will make your prayer to Him, He will hear you, and you will pay your vows. You will also declare a thing, and it will be established for you; so light will shine on your ways. Job 22:27-28

Rick was relapsing. Dialysis caused him to go downhill. He said he'd rather be dead than take dialysis and he wished he was dead. He complained before every dialysis treatment, so I went in on him this morning, "Do not talk like that, you are so negative, God knows your thoughts, and He knows everything about you. Move out of your own way, move out of God's way, stop blocking your blessings, recovery and healing. Satan can cause divine chastisement and it has eternal consequences. Sin is disobedience to God and He hates sin because of what it does to his creation, his children.

Satan is a destroyer, divider, deceives, disappoints, makes big time offers that it cannot fulfill, makes awesome promises, it cannot produce, temporary satisfaction, destructive, destroys families, marriages, children, and sin brings sickness and death, sometimes sudden but the worst thing is eternal fire from Satan. At least with God, you get eternal life. The blood of Jesus Christ is your saving grace. The price of sin is blood. You keep putting limitations on what you can do. There is no limitation on what God can do. God did not give you a stroke. God did not cause your kidneys to fail, and it's not God's fault that you did not take care of yourself, God has given you another chance and you're still not taking advantage of that, you do not take care of you, you rely on me to take care of you, and you need to take special care of yourself, especially being a diabetic and a stroke survivor. God is still willing to heal you, you have all your faculties, and all your limbs, so focus, think positive, and put death to rest, out of your mind, focus totally on living. Trust God to heal you and if that is not His will, allow Him to help you endure it to the end for however short or long the end may be! Keep the faith and never lose hope. If you are dying, you are wasting precious time because you are not dead yet."

I call heaven and earth as witnesses today against you, that I have set before your life and death, blessing and cursing; therefore choose life, that both you and your descendants may live. Deuteronomy 30:19

I exclaimed that it wasn't the sickness that wanted him to die. He felt powerless, but he had the power to take control of his health and he did not have to do it alone. He had God and me, but he kept allowing that sick weak spirit to creep in and attack his well spirit and his will to live. His mindset was shifting back and forth between a bad day to dooms day. Rick was waiting for the end, waiting to die, planning on dying. Most days, I was exhausted and merely going through the motion of caring for a baby in a man's body. He was my big baby. After all, I created that monster. "Pray," I said, "God really does answer prayers so keep praying and never give up."

Therefore I say to you, whatever things you ask when you pray, believe that you receive them, and you will have them. Mark 11:24

I was at his place more than my own now, so I had pretty much moved into his apartment at this point although it was against my better judgment. God was guiding me and giving me the strength to do what I needed to do, and it had nothing to do with what I wanted. When God guides you to do something, you do not question it, you just do it, so I rolled with the flow. Rick was wheelchair dependent now, but in good spirits, and he loved sitting out front with neighbors while I prepared dinner.

I can do all things through Christ who strengthens me. Philippians 4:13

Rick still hated dialysis, but he was doing well, no more strokes, congested heart failures, he had not been hospitalized in quite a while, and his lab reports were very good. He was well on his way to becoming an end renal disease survivor.

Seeing their faith, Jesus said to the paralyzed man, "My child, your sins are forgiven." Mark 2:5

Suddenly, I began noticing something strange and different. Rick appeared confused. When I spoke to the doctors about it, they attributed it to a side effect from one or several of the many medications he was taking, as well as the kidney disease, so I left it alone. Once I arrive at home, I started going through all his bottles of medicines to see what the various side effects were. Two of them listed memory loss. At the beginning, he would even catch himself saying or doing something ridiculous or that didn't make any sense, so the fact that he would catch himself at times made me think he was still pretty much in control of it, mentally. He would mention it, shake his head, laugh and sometimes even apologize. I knew that his sickness was not going to mysteriously go away, but I sure didn't want him to get any worse. In addition, I wanted him to realize that he really didn't want to die until it was his time, but I knew he was sick of being sick and he didn't need anything else going wrong. The thought of being on dialysis made him sick. I was confident that God is a healer and I had seen God's miracles several times, once was when He healed my fibromyalgia (over 30 years ago) and during a time when doctors had no idea how to treat the agonizing and excruciating pain that shot from my head to my toes, so I knew from experience that prayer has worked even when medicine fails. Another time was when a longtime friend tested negative to HIV after 25 years of suffering with the disease. I know a male who was healed of herpies after 20 years. Rick knew my faith was strong, so I reiterated to him: "My God is in the healing and lifesaving business and I must do God's work, I'm a vessel, that's all I am, so all you need to do is allow God to do His will, God wants to change your heart, heal your body, and spirit, you are a real sweetheart but that's not enough to get you into heaven."

I will give you a new heart and put a new spirit in you; I will remove your heart of stone and give you a heart of flesh. And I will put my Spirit in you and move you to follow my decrees and be careful to keep my laws. Ezekiel 36:26-27

He was looking at me like I was crazy but at least I had his undivided attention. "Follow my lead," I said, "God is like oxygen, you cannot see it, but you cannot live without it. Like God, you cannot see Him, and you can't live without Him either." Rick had to believe, and he had to be saved. God was always putting words in my mouth and I thank Him because most of the time I was lost for words. "Even in your weakest moments," I continued, "you can be strong because God's grace is all you have and need." He was quiet and focusing all his attention on me. He was listening without interrupting me. I could feel his desire to get his spirit and health back. I could detect his fear of death as well. At this moment, I knew I would never give up on him.

God is committed to us so never stop striving, instead allow God's supernatural grace to carry us, it will empower us to naturally carry out God's "good work."

He asked, "How does God empower us?" I replied, "By giving us a new heart and spirit, a new heart of Jesus inside us. God's Spirit continually gives us the grace (yearning and authority) to do what is pleasing to Him. His grace is the voice that calls us to change and the power to be victorious and although the bible was written a gazillion years ago, we must think of God as doing it now to be a conqueror. To tap into God's good grace, we must believe and trust God. Prayer is the olive branch that moves us in the direction of grace. What gets in the way is being an unbeliever and that change is going to happen when it's going to happen."

If any of you lacks wisdom, let him ask of God, who gives to all liberally and without reproach, and it will be given to him. But let him ask in faith, with no doubting, for he who doubts is like a wave of the sea driven and tossed by the wind. For let not that man suppose that he will receive anything from the Lord; he is a double-minded man, unstable in all his ways. James 1:5-8

Wow, Rick said, "Yeah, what's the point of praying if we don't believe or trust in God? I answered, "There comes a point in your life when you must surrender and stop trying to do things on your own and trust that God's goodness is enough." Rick not only needed physical help, he also needed his spirit renewed so I ended the conversation with, "Grace motivates me, and it is given not because we have done good works, but in order that we may be able to do them and one sure way to get your life back is by God's good grace.

Therefore if anyone cleanses himself from the latter, he will be a vessel for honor, sanctified and useful for the Master, prepared for every good work. 2 Timothy 2:21

Basically, Rick's life had been easy, so this was the big test and the first time in his life that he was not in control, lost in the sauce. Up to this point, everything in his life was good. His bad marriages, the death of his mom, dad, or brother couldn't compare to what he was going through, dialysis, stroke survivor, in need of a kidney transplant, fighting for his life, and wondering how much longer he had on this earth. Rick was like a rebellious teenager when it came to God. It was time for him to surrender.

Therefore we do not lose heart. Even though our outward man is perishing, yet the inward man is being renewed day by day. For our light affliction, which is but for a moment, is working for us a far more exceeding and eternal weight of glory, while we do not look at the things which are seen, but at the things which are not seen. For the things which are seen are temporary, but the things which are not seen are eternal. 2 Corinthians 4:16-18

God could make him strong if he would just trust Him so I constantly recited scripture after scripture in hopes of giving him a constant shot of Jesus throughout the day every day.

Grace is the power of God's love drawing us and enabling us to respond to Him.

Scriptures kept me strong, so I thought they could do the same for him. I tried to tell him in no uncertain terms that the only way to deal with sickness was to trust in God's promises and if he rejects God's offer and promises to help, there is no hope for mercy from God. It was in his best interest to develop a close relationship with God. It was hard to tell a meathead how to get close to God. When I was lost for words, I would just say, "read the bible, all the answers are in the bible with all of God's promises and principles too. It will comfort you. You must ask to receive. Pray."

63

*These things I have spoken to you, that in Me you may have
peace. In the world you will have tribulation; but be of good
cheer, I have overcome the world. John 16:33*

"I'm going to try to make the best of a bad situation and be
strong," Rick said, "it could always be worst." I held and
rubbed his hands as I recited one of my favorite quotes,
"When God leads you to the edge of the cliff, trust Him fully
and let go because he'll either catch you, teach you how to
fly, or carry you, but he will never let you fall, so trust Him."
I had faith that God was working on him. He was dozing
off. When he fell asleep, I prayed, "He's yours, Lord, please
empty all the old out of him, and renew his spirit and restore
his health, give Rick the will to live, transform him, align all
his organs to work in perfect order, if anyone can do it, You
can. You created his body; you can heal his body. Forgive
us all, Lord, for our sins. I pray that it be your will to give
Rick the trust and strength he needs to simply cope and be
saved so that he can rest in paradise, eternally. Thank you,
Father, In the name of Jesus, Amen."

*I will say of the LORD, "He is my refuge and my fortress; My
God, in Him I will trust." Psalm 91:2*

It can be extremely overwhelming when there's no hope that
your loved one will ever get better. But, I had to remain
optimistic because it was my job to show Rick how God
really works in my life and how He can work in his. A lot
of people felt that I was in denial, but he wasn't dead so why
shouldn't I be optimistic? I choose to be strong and if I'm in
denial, then denial was helping me to pace my feelings and
gave me a certain amount of poise. It is God's way of not
giving me anymore than I could take because Rick and I may
have been taken by surprise, but nothing takes God by
surprise, and I knew that God would not allow this situation

64

to overwhelm us as long as we stayed focused and looked to Him.

We're put here on Earth to learn our own lessons. No one can tell you what your lessons are; it is part of your personal journey to discover them. On these journeys we may be given a lot, or just a little bit of the things we must grapple with, but never more than we can handle. Dr. Elisabeth Kubler-Ross

I knew that God's guidance and blessings always outweighed any of my struggles or troubles. I just did not know how to convey this to Rick who had his doubts even though he knew God had answered many of my prayers and many of his too. He was a very sick man who just wanted to take the easy way out. He had about enough faith the size of a tiny mustard seed which is all he needed.

So Jesus said to them, "Because of your unbelief; for assuredly, I say to you, if you have faith as a mustard seed, you will say to this mountain, 'Move from here to there,' and it will move; and nothing will be impossible for you." Matthew 17:20

Rick could not understand for the life of him why he would have a stroke that would leave him with right-side weakness and wheelchair bound when he knew people who were way worse individuals than him. I explained to him that a lot of people have it all, they live like the devil, and although they have every material thing in the world, when it comes to facing pain, suffering, struggling or hard times, they don't have jack, no strength, no God, no power, nothing. This is when some people find God because it takes courage to go through difficulties, pain and suffering. He felt he did not deserve to have a stroke. Regardless, to what he felt, he had a stroke, and he had to deal with it. I encouraged him to stop comparing his life to others and focus on Jesus who is a healer, to keep the faith, and never give up. "You'd be surprised what the Holy Spirit can do for you," to you, and with you." "During difficult times, God gives you the courage, strength, confidence, boldness, and readiness to face life," I said, "again, sometimes bad things happen to good people, it's life and sometimes life really sucks."

. . . teaching in their synagogues, preaching the gospel of the kingdom, and healing all kinds of sickness and all kinds of disease among the people. Matthew 4:23

I needed just as much help as Rick. I needed a shoulder to cry on myself sometimes. I finally began to realize that the man I'd grown to love and know for all these years, a sport's enthusiast, diehard Redskin fan as well as a Pittsburgh Steelers fan, who had a real knack for cooking, entertaining, hard-worker, homebody, fun, loving, sweetheart of a man suddenly needed more than a partner, a wife, lover and friend. There was a lot that I had to face and admit. I had to accept the fact that my perfect gentleman, my Knight and shiny armor, my Prince charming needed a hospital bed and a permanent nurse. I questioned myself, "Am I in denial?" I thought to myself, "He's still alive but he has no real quality of life. After all these years, he still can't transfer himself from the wheelchair to the bed, chair or sofa." If he hadn't stopped physical and occupational therapy, he could do more. Occupational therapy would have helped with dressing himself and physical therapy would have helped him to transfer himself and kept him strong physically or it may have helped him to avoid the wheelchair altogether had he not stopped. We'll never know. The reality was that the love of my life and my best friend was dying. That was the first time I said it aloud. It's been in the back of my head for years but now it was in the forefront of my mind. OOG (Oh Our God!), I put my head in my hands. I couldn't breathe, I was hyperventilating, my legs were heavy, my stomach was queasy, my nose was running, I was crying, my knees felt swollen and tight, and my head was pounding. I kept inhaling and exhaling, breathing in and out. I had to breathe; I had to make myself breathe. I could not get it out of my head, "Rick is really dying, oh no, Rick is dying. I felt like I was suffocating." My stomach went from queasy to aching. I was so emotional, nauseated, and bent over. It had finally hit me, and hit me hard that Rick was dying. I ran to the bathroom to put water on my face and threw up. I boohooed until I almost passed out. I fell to the floor, banging and crying.

But Jesus turned around, and when He saw her He said, "Be of good cheer, daughter; your faith has made you well." And the woman was made well from that hour. Matthew 9:22

I had to pull it together. God gives us the authority and power to empower or disempower and unfortunately, Rick was stuck on "I can't do it," but not me, I wasn't stuck on anything but Jesus. He felt as though he couldn't do anything and that I could do it all although I could only do but so much. He said I was his eyes, ears, arms, legs, his everything. He needed to get the word "can't" out of his vocabulary. Don't get me wrong, this was a real huge pill for me to swallow too. I didn't want to lose my man, my best friend, the best man I ever had, plus he was just way too young to die. Not that it was up to me, but I wasn't ready for him to die. Not yet, anyway and the thought of losing him made me think twice and feel somewhat guilty about the time we wasted being apart when I wasn't ready to take care of him. I could not stop thinking about the fact that Rick could really die. There sure isn't any way to prepare for death except arrange his funeral and wait for his expiration date. Is there a proper way to respond to death? If Rick didn't get anything else, he got the fact that he was going to die, he got that a long time ago, but he got stuck on death. I didn't quite get it, I wasn't claiming it, and I didn't want to believe it, but I could not be in denial any longer. I also didn't want to be on death watch. Although it had been happening for years, I still didn't want to believe that this was happening to us, that Rick was going to die. I was an emotional wreck, but I had to come to my senses, we're all going to die one day and in the meantime, we must keep the faith because God gives us the authority to press forward with determination and conviction.

Grace and peace be multiplied to you in the knowledge of God and of Jesus our Lord, as His divine power has given to us all things that pertain *to life and godliness, through the knowledge of Him who called us by glory and virtue, by which have been given to us exceedingly great and precious promises, that through these you may be partakers of the divine nature, having escaped the corruption* that is *in the world through lust. 2 Peter 1:4*

Grace does not come without struggle, but it does promise the presence of God. He's your father, loving you unconditionally and you are one of His many defiant children, so He continues to extend his grace. This is a transformation, a new lifestyle and lifetime mission, so be patience with yourself because it is not going to happen overnight. God will change you if you allow Him and His grace will form your life.

God knows our weaknesses, He created our bodies and He will complete His work inside of us if we let him.

God is the designer and God is fitting you for a purpose. We're all a work in progress and while my faith is unwavering Rick wasn't there yet and fighting for one's life is probably the toughest and worse fight anyone can ever have. I just wanted Rick to be a happy sick man and find contentment. It was a heavy blow for me too, but I trust God because if we trust Him he will transform us.

I knew that I couldn't save him but the caregiving nature and the God in me was telling me otherwise. He didn't want to live after the stroke but he's still alive. I reminded him, "You are not a stroke victim or statistic, rather you are a stroke survivor, now get that through your thick skull and praise God instead of feeling sorry for yourself." Rick had been sick for years. He was a typical sick person, up and down with his emotions, good and bad days, but in good spirits most days. The medication he was on was keeping him heavily sedated and he loved it. He was content, very comfortable, feeling no pain. He was peaceful and quiet. I was praying without ceasing and God was answering my prayers more and more and it was the God in me giving me the strength to get through each day. Listening to music soothed his demeanor and watching sports kept him entertained and interested. Personally, I felt that television overall wasn't stimulating enough for his mind, but I went along with whatever kept him quiet and in a good mood. If he had a good day, then I had a wonderful day. It wasn't about me.

I cried to Him with my mouth, and He was extolled with my tongue. If I regard iniquity in my heart, the Lord will not hear. But certainly God has heard me; He has attended to the voice of my prayer. Blessed be God, who has not turned away my prayer, nor His mercy from me! Psalm 66:17-20

Rick never understood the severity dialysis, or he just didn't care because the dialysis treatments had completely stopped the congestive heart failures, reduced the blood transfusions, and fluid retention a whole lot so it was working, but he still complained every time he had to go to dialysis. "I'm too weak"; "it races my heart"; "they almost lost me the last time." No matter what, he was still alive, and dialysis was a necessity. Just like with physical and occupational therapies, he made one complaint after another. I told him, "As long as you can open your eyes, you are going to dialysis—life is what you make it and if you want to play God, you go right ahead and if you don't go to dialysis you will surely die. It's your life and your choice. You make the call, dialysis or death? I cannot choose for you or make you want to live if you keep insisting that you want to die, but no problem is too great for my God and wherever you are in your life you can die off from what you were and become anew and it's never too late to change. God can transform you, if you would just give him a chance."

And do not be conformed to this world, but be transformed by the renewing of your mind, that you may prove what is good and acceptable and perfect will of God. Romans 12:2

"I will say it a gazillion times 'you need Jesus so trust Him', that's all you need to do. Love yourself. Change your mind and you will change your behavior and if there is no room for change there is no room for growth. Believe in the power of God and His power to heal, believe He is a way-maker, and He will make a way out of no way for you just like he does for me. God is going to give me the strength and the tools to help you, but you got to believe, and you need to show God that you trust Him. It's hard enough watching someone fight for their life but to give up doesn't make any sense at all. I just want you to be able to receive God's mercy." "I trust Him, I honestly do," Rick said reassuringly.

But now God has shown us a different way of being right in his sight—not by obeying the law but by the way promised in the Scriptures long ago. We are made right in God's sight when we trust in Jesus Christ to take away our sins. And we all can be saved in this same way, no matter who we are or what we have done. Romans 3:21-22

"All you have to do is expect that God is going to restore your health," I continued, "put you out of your misery, just put your focus and energy on the Lord, "pray and ask Him to forgive your sins, ask for help, ask Jesus to guide you, direct your path for you. If you don't want to talk to Him or know how to pray, merely call His name, call on Jesus, call on God. If you do not take sin seriously, recognizing every time you've come before God asking for forgiveness, He shed His blood for all people everywhere and sin is serious, so serious it caused God his only begotten son. Jesus died on the cross so that we could have a relationship with God, God's love has no end. He atoned for the sin of the entire world. The bible is about what's coming and what's coming again. If you come to grips with your sinning lifestyle and want to be forgiven, God will show you His will. If it hasn't happened yet, one thing you don't want to do is die before it does. Why should you doubt Him? If you doubt him then what? People have feelings of unworthiness, but we are all equally loved by God so God is equally active in all of lives, He loves us all the same, the closer we are to him the more we are going to receive, he does not play favoritism. Peter, Paul and John had a better relationship with God than most. He doesn't love anyone more than he loves you. He is the only one that can get you to heaven, He died on your behalf, so you don't have to die in sin. Pick up the bible, God is the heart of the gospel that will get you into heaven.

And if you call on the Father, who without partiality judges according to each one's work, conduct yourself throughout the time of your stay here in fear; knowing that you were not redeemed with corruptible things, like silver or gold, from your aimless conduct received by tradition from your fathers, but was the precious blood of Christ, as of a lamb without blemish and without spot. He indeed was foreordained before the foundation of the world, but was manifest in these times for you who through Him believe in God, who raised Him from the dead and gave Him glory, so that your faith and hope are in God. 1 Peter 1:17-21

Personally, I love Psalm, Isaiah, Jeremiah and Proverbs, just pick up your bible, dust it off, open it and read it. Your whole eternal future may depend on the blood of Jesus and if you do not know where to start, start with the new testament (Matthew, Mark, Luke, John). God already knows your heart and all your needs and when you read it to yourself, aloud, you'll get what I've been saying." The Holy Spirit is deep, and you can feel the presence of God.

And suddenly there came a sound from heaven, as of a rushing mighty wind, and it filled the whole house where they were sitting. Then there appeared to them divided tongues, as of fire, and one sat upon each of them. And they were all filled with the Holy Spirit and began to speak with other tongues, as the Spirit gave them utterance. Acts 2:2-4

I recalled a "not weak" scripture my granny taught me as a kid that stuck in my head like a hymn:

Praise the LORD, O my soul, and forget not all his benefits who forgives all your sins and heals all your diseases; who redeems your life from the pit and crowns you with love and compassion; who satisfies your desires with good things so that your youth is renewed like the eagles. Psalm 103:2-5

"Seek all your answers from the Lord, Rick," I said, "those who seek God shall find Him. You need to relax in His presence, rely on His promises, and trust in His timing. Things may not happen when you want them to, but they are happening. You are like a withered plant, but you still have a lot of life in you. You are not dead yet." He smiled and cried, "Touch and agree, you always perk me up, but I like the way you said that. If anyone can make me want to live,

it's you, you are one in a trillion and I couldn't do this
without you," he boohooed, "you are my earth angel." I said,
"All glory be to God, we couldn't do this without Jesus,
without God, and thank God we have each other and are
surrounded by angels." He started singing, "Take me to the
river, drop me in the water." I loved it when he was in a
singing mood and feeling hopeful.

*"Come to Me, all you who labor [are weary] and are heavy
laden [carrying heavy burdens], and I will give you rest.
Take My yoke upon you and learn from Me, for I am gentle
and lowly in heart, and you will find rest for your souls. For
My yoke is easy and My burden is light." Matthew 11:28-
30*

I tried to explain to Rick that hope is endless and you cannot
cope without hope. He was too sweet not to have more faith.
I encouraged him to cling to hope to keep him from slipping
into a dark place again. Although he was sick, he was not as
bad he used to be. However, I was concerned about the
confusion. Rick occupied all my time and sometimes I felt
like I was in solitary confinement but his complements, love,
appreciation and being called a "wonderful wife," a "good
and kind hearted woman" somehow made it all worthwhile.
He was very appreciative.

*Houses and riches are an inheritance from fathers,
But a prudent wife is from the LORD. Proverbs 19:14*

My father was a peaceful man who taught me as a kid to
"take the good with the bad; the bitter with the sweet; the
word 'can't' wasn't a part of my vocabulary; never give up;
never settle for less; and it could always be worse." None of

that made as much sense then as it does now. "When God made you, He was showing off," is how my father raised my siblings and me so we grew up with extremely high self-esteem, over confident and believing "we could do anything; nothing beats a failure but a try; there are consequences to your actions; karma is a bitch; you get out of life what you put into it, if you put nothing in, you'll get nothing out; the moon is the limit, and if you do something wrong, just don't get caught." My mom and dad pumped all of us up all the time and encouraged us to be all we could be. My mom said I was 10 years old when I was born so I have always been mature for my age. They taught us that there wasn't anything that we couldn't do if we put our minds to it, and best of all "sticks and stones may break your bones, but words should never hurt you." I love and appreciate my parents for equipping me with tough skin and the ability to take on challenges with conviction and determination. The main thing is to never give up.

Let us not become weary in doing good, for at the proper time we will reap a harvest if we do not give up. Galatians 6:9

I tried to keep Rick focused on all the good times we had. Just getting through the day wasn't enough, I had to find a way to keep him encouraged amid this storm the best way I could. We spoke about him joining a support group so that he could get back to his old self, but he wasn't interested at all. "Patience," I kept telling myself! Rick was already feeling bad enough, so I didn't want to do anything to discourage him anymore than he already was. I was talking to myself more and more lately because there wasn't anyone else to talk to. I was not a complainer, but I was tired all the time and hungry all the time, so I had plenty to complain about. Food was very comforting. Before, Rick was chilled and laid back with not a care in the world. We agreed to disagree if we had any differences of opinions. I had my own bank account and he had his. We have never argued over money or anything in the past but now all we do is argue about what he's not doing to get better. We really loved, communicated and respected each other so we had no disagreements and even now, if he would just do what he needed to do to get healthier or better we would be great. He's just spoiled and stubborn. I was not willing to spend the rest of my life with a man who gave up a long time ago and who has no quality of life. I just wasn't going to put myself in that predicament.

Beareth all things, believeth all things, hopeth all things, endureth all things. 1 Corinthians 13:7

Rick hated dialysis because it was a form of life support, I get that, and he never wanted to be on any type of life support, I get that, and I can't blame him for that. I knew he was going to die, and so was I, eventually. But, he isn't dead yet, so live life to your fullest until you die, but he was living to die, and on constant death watch. What was that about? We all know our birthdate, but no one knows their expiration date. I didn't want to think about it either, I could go before him, the one the sickest doesn't always go the quickest. He was dwelling on death so hard he began having dreams and nightmares about dead people, family members, friends, ghosts and scary looking clowns, so we talked about death a lot. We simply took it one day at a time. Rick was a work in progress, praise God. I prayed night and day that the Lord would deliver us.

When the righteous cry for help, the Lord hears and delivers them out of all their troubles. Psalm 34:17

Whether Rick liked dialysis or not, it was his lifeline, and keeping him alive. He had to be strong and keep the faith. He was burdening himself with dying again. Rick was going to have to reach way down and get some strength from somewhere or that sick spirit was going to overtake him again and again and again. He needed to stay strong, let go and let God.

If you fail under pressure, your strength is not very great. Proverbs 24:10

Rick said that he did not want to take dialysis because he did not want to be sick for the rest of his life. Whether he took dialysis or not, he probably was going to be sick for the rest of his life because the stroke affected his brain and nervous system. "Please stop living to die and stop making death seem so awful, and again death is a part of life and death ends a life not a relationship." He laughed and said, "Wow," 'stop living to die, and death ends a life, not a relationship' hmmm, food for thought because that's exactly what I've been doing, Lord have mercy, you're right, I need to stop talking about dying and just let it happen when it happens instead of constantly making it a bad thing. You're right, I'm still alive! Who knows how much longer it's going to be, look how long it's been already and I haven't gone anywhere yet. You are absolutely right." He was finally getting it, I think, finally believing, "dying was a part of life and not so bad after all." I sure hope so. We both smiled and kissed. It was a relief. Hallelujah! At least he was not on death watch tonight or living to die. Praise the Lord! Thank you, Jesus!

Call upon me in the day of trouble; I will deliver you, and you shall glorify me. Psalm 50:15

I was exhausted mentally and physically. You know what keeps me up, I'm under obligation, I'm committed to the Lord. I absolutely cherished a peaceful night. Rick had me feeling like a yoyo with all his ups and downs, more downs than ups. I was tired, and it was the same old thing repeatedly. He constantly complained about not wanting to do dialysis. I knew it took a lot out of him, but I would ignore him, dress him, and take him there anyway. I would download dialysis success stories but none of that mattered to him. When he went to dialysis, he never wanted to complete his treatment and would ask to end his treatment early. His time had already been reduced 15 minutes. Rick often gave me a hard time, but I was time enough for him. I felt bad for the nurses and technicians especially when I stepped out of the treatment area to use the bathroom, get something to eat and/or drink. Thank God, he basically did anything that I told him to do, but not without some lip action, he was sassy, stubborn and spoiled. I had gotten good with turning him off and on. Nothing he said mattered if he stayed on the machine for his entire treatment. I am so guilty of spoiling him, it was merely my great adoration and expression of my love for him, perhaps an expression of too much love. We had no idea what was going on, but I was told by his kidney and primary care doctors that the blood wasn't flowing fast enough from his feet, to his heart, to his brain; he's a stroke survivor; side effects from meds, plus he was on dialysis. No matter what, I still loved him, I just didn't know how much more I could take but I knew by the grace of God that I would survive and endure it to the end. I just didn't know if it was going to be his end or my end.

Above all, love each other deeply, because love covers over a multitude of sins. 1 Peter 4:8

I was working as a legal assistant by day and a caregiver by night. I had an attitude because I was exhausted all the time. Thank God, I didn't suffer with depression, but I started taking some St. John's Wort anyway because I was too tired to think sometimes. I had not been to the doctor's in years, so I have no idea what I was suffering with. I was just tired and saying it at this point meant absolutely nothing to anyone anymore because it was nothing anyone could do to help. He was way too far gone to be left with anyone except a qualified and skillful nurse. We were on our own. I relentlessly prayed, "Give me strength." I thanked God for getting me through another rough day, day-after-day. Oftentimes, I felt as though I was sleep-walking. My body was here but I don't know where my mind was. I really didn't like this feeling of perplexity and all I wanted was a good night's sleep.

We are pressed on every side by troubles, but we are not crushed. We are perplexed, but not driven to despair. We are hunted down, but never abandoned by God. We get knocked down, but we are not destroyed. 1 Corinthians 4:8

I had a good night's sleep, but it was obvious Rick didn't. I woke up praising the Lord and he awakes complaining, as usual, "Why me Lord?" He was really upset about waking up this morning. It was my new normal and every day I was faced with giving him a faith-lift which kept me strong and for the most part, kept us both in good spirits or as well as could be expected considering the circumstances and all that we were going through. "The nerve of you to question God about anything, why not you, Rick," I asked, "would you rather it be one of your children or grandchildren, someone else you have in mind?" He looked real dumbfounded and sounded mad when he replied, "To be honest, I wish it wasn't me, but I wouldn't wish my life on my worst forking enemy." Shaking my head, I said, "You are allowing your sickness to destroy your life, and moving forward you need to humble yourself. You are running away from life, and it really sounds like you have a death wish, you are doing everything, except trying to live. There is a time and place for everything, death will come soon enough, so live until it does, today is the time to live. You are alive, not dead for the umpteenth time. It certainly sounds like you'd rather be dead. Be careful what you ask for, God just might answer your prayers and grant you your wish. Why are you so angry and bitter though? You make me not want to be around you. God and love are the only things that will get us through this." He apologized, hugged, kissed and thanked me. He promised to do better. I was not going to hold my breath, but I wanted him to feel good before I left him for the day, so I bathed, shaved, washed his hair, lotion him down, massaged his back legs, arms, dressed, and cooked breakfast. Before we ate we prayed: "Heavenly Father, thank you for another day to get it right. Thank you for waking us up this morning. Great things come to those who are patient and don't give up, better things come to those who believe in, and trust God and the best things come to those who are obedient and never give up. I know that you're a teacher, doctor, lawyer, healer, prophet, and most of all our Lord and Savior and that we are all your children. Give us strength, endurance, constant compassion and patience to power forward. Guide Rick to a happy place in his life and show him how to rest in your presence while you are restoring his health, and renewing his spirit. We would like to thank you for my health. We thank you for the challenges. Thank you for the food we eat, the clothes we wear, and the home we live in. We ask that you cover us all, family, friends, neighbors, children and grandchildren in the blood of Jesus and that you continue to protect us all from evil. In the Name of Your Son, Christ Jesus, Amen.

But if we walk in the light as He is in the light, we have fellowship with one another, and the blood of Jesus Christ His Son cleanses us from all sin. If we say that we have no sin, we deceive ourselves, and the truth is not in us. If we confess our sins, He is faithful and just to forgive us our sins and to cleanse us from all unrighteousness. 1 John 1:7-9

God bless America and God bless the world. Bless our children and our streets. Thank you for your favor and for blessing us abundantly, Lord, there would be no us if it weren't for you. Bless Rick to encounter Your love and trust, impact his heart and mind, so that he can reap the benefits of your blessons and deliverance. Guide him to live for You and not for himself. Show him that God's love is chasing him down and that 'goodness and mercy shall follow him all the days of his life,' if he trusts You. In the Name of Your Son, Christ Jesus, Amen." He cosigned, "Amen, Amen, Amen. Thank you, that was a lovely and powerful prayer. Lord, have mercy on me. Forgive me for all my sins. God bless you. I needed and received that, and I feel so good, full and clean. You know I love a bath." "I know," I said, "you used to take two to three showers a day during the summertime. Ain't nothing wrong with that, cleanliness is next to godliness."

Cleanliness is next to Godliness. Acts 9:32-10:23

"Do not tell me that 'cleanliness is next to Godliness' is in the Bible," Rick said. I gestured my head, yes, and as we ate, we talked, laughed and enjoyed reminiscing about our "Soap" tapes with Billy Crystal playing a gay guy. Rick literally had me rolling on the floor laughing, marking the characters. Soap was hysterical and helped us to laugh our way through some really difficult times. I would take a laugh every chance I got, so any old excuse to laugh was good enough for me. He was happy, smiling, joking, and in a better mood than when he woke up and that's all that mattered. I really didn't know how to fix someone so broken and who was living to die so I was blessed to see him in an exceptionally good mood before I left him for the day. Prayer was working! God was working upfront and behind the scenes, one day at a time. Glory, glory, hallelujah!

For nothing is impossible with God. Luke 1:37

Time was getting away from me and I'll be totally exhausted when I do get to work but the look on his face and his disposition, this morning, was priceless. I wheeled him from the dining room back into the bedroom. He looked so good for such a sick man. Rick ate good and I really enjoyed our morning together. Wishful thinking, I prayed that every morning could be like this. Thank you, Lord for an amazingly joyful start to my day.

I slept and I dreamed that life is all joy. I woke and I saw that life is all service. I served and I saw that service is joy.
Khalil Gibran

Before going out the door, he commented about being happy, uplifted and feeling the Holy Spirit. I was proud of him. "Keep seeking God's love because His love is personal," I said, "get to know God on an intimate and friendly level, God's love is focused on each one of us, God knows you, God loves you, God is hyperconscious of you, God is elated when you are happy and smiling. Even when you cry, like I said before, God collects your tears in a bottle and has them all numbered, God takes note of every tear you shed and knows what brought on those tears, so God is both universal, omnipresent, everywhere, all the time and personal, caring for you individually. God's love is not antagonistic, it's friendly and tremendously supportive. He loves every person as if they were the only person in the world to love."

For God so loved the world that He gave His only begotten Son, that whoever believes in Him should not perish but have everlasting life. John 3:16

Love was in the air. What a blessing? I could go to work, in peace, and leave him in good spirits. Praise God. Rick was living in the now and he was pleasant to be around especially this morning. That was a relief. I spoke to him throughout the day and he was still up and in a great mood. When I returned home that evening he was playing solitary on my laptop in a cheerful mood. He said he had drank a little of my red wine and sent his children an email. He wasn't computer savvy, so both the computer and wine were unfamiliar territory and out of the ordinary for him. He used email, very seldom, and only at work so he was not a computer or email user at all. He called the wine "liquid courage" and sounded relieved and pleased because he had gotten some things off his chest regarding his children. He drank an occasional Corona, maybe once a month so it probably did him some good to drink a little red wine. Even the bible says we should.

Don't drink only water. You ought to drink a little wine for the sake of your stomach because you are sick so often. 1 Timothy 5:23

He stayed up much longer than usual, playing Chess, Yahtzee and Dominoes. I was gamed out. As I watched the sunset, I couldn't help but to think about how much time Rick spent on such insignificant issues. My thoughts were interrupted when he came outside to watch the sunset too. I was happy to see him so energized. Afterwards, I nodded in and out as I sat in the chair and he watched television and played Mrs. Pacman before he crashed for the night. He was exercising and using his nerve damaged hand more. I give him an "e" for effort, at least he was trying, today. He had a full day and so did I. "Praise the Lord, it was a good day."

Praise him for his mighty acts: praise him according to his excellent greatness. Praise him with the sound of the trumpet: praise him with the psaltery and harp. Praise him with the timbrel and dance: praise him with stringed instruments and organs. Praise him upon the loud cymbals: praise him upon the high sounding cymbals. Let everything that hath breath praise the LORD. Praise ye the LORD. Psalm 150:2-6

The next morning, he woke in a marvelous mood. We talked a lot and I explained further about asking God to help him with his weaknesses, that God is a burden-bearer, and He doesn't expect us to take on these types of things alone. We prayed that his children would show him some love, a simple telephone call would suffice, and that's basically all he wanted.

Give your burdens to the Lord, and he will take care of you. He will not permit the godly to slip and fall. Psalm 55:22

Most of the dialysis patients' caregivers complained about their loved one's lack of sleep, talking in their sleep, and dementia (screaming, hollering, and memory loss). I prayed that our love was strong enough to endure that challenge because I had begun noticing that Rick was showing more and more signs of confusion, memory loss and symptoms of dementia. Dementia patients required way more caregiving than normal. Therefore, I wasn't looking forward to taking care of a dementia patient, someone who would eventually forget me. Right now, he was sleeping pretty good, so I'll cross that bridge when I get there but in the meantime, we will be trying to pray dementia away. The thought of dementia was scary. I prayed God takes my dementia fears away.

There is no fear in love. But perfect love drives out fear because fear has to do with punishment. The one who fears is not made perfect in love. We love because he first loved us. 1 John 4:18-19

After a while Rick was amazed that I could backup everything that I said with a bible scripture and I was happy that he realized that before he lost his memory completely. I was making a true believer out of him, after all. I think that's what God intended. I began to realize that it wasn't about me at all, but about Jesus and Rick getting to know Jesus and his salvation. I asked myself, "Lord have mercy, was I chosen to preach the gospel to Rick?" I could hear God's voice, "Come, and follow me!"

God knows best, He makes no mistakes, lead, I will definitely follow.

Rick and I talked about focusing on going to heaven. He really didn't want to live but he was taking things in stride now and concentrating more on living than dying and that was a good thing. He was doing a balancing act between the light and the dark side but leaning more towards the light. I just wanted him to live while he was alive. Death was already coming soon enough. I was only human, merely a goodhearted woman, I was not a miracle worker therefore aside from providing the care of giving, TLC, encouragement, prayer, nutrition, and help with his salvation, what more could I do when he gave up a long time ago?

Give all your worries and cares to God for He cares about you. 1 Peter 5:7

I could feel a blessing coming, not defeat, a healing, and deliverance. "Believe that God is releasing goodness over your life, a healing over your life," I said, "blessing your life, and giving you another chance at life. He wants to release a flood of His power over you, and anoint your life. God is a conqueror! Dare to believe; flip the switch, turn life on and death off – flip from doubt and fear to faith and meditate thinking about God's favor, grace, mercy, and love and don't think about how long you've been sick but that every day is a blessing because you survived another day, you are a survivor." Even if it doesn't turn out the way you expected or wanted it to, at least you did not spend your last days dwelling on death, instead choosing to live your best life ever despite your health prognosis.

He will take these weak mortal bodies of ours and change them into glorious bodies like his own, using the same mighty power that he will use to conquer everything everywhere. Philippians 3:21

We had a great dinner and evening. I talked him to sleep so I was able to chillax early. Sweet dreams, my love. I took pleasure in overindulging in a slice of strawberry shortcake, with ice cream, carmel syrup, and extra whip cream. God really does know how much a person can take. Praise Him! It was a joyful and peaceful night. Thank you, Lord. Good looking out!

Therefore do not worry about tomorrow, for tomorrow will worry about itself. Each day has enough trouble of its own. Matthew 6:34

Every day is the day that the Lord has made. I took every day, one day at a time because our lives were so unpredictable. This morning Rick woke with a bad attitude, complaining about dialysis, nothing unusual since this was the norm to the start of his dialysis days. "I'm never going to dialysis again, I quit," he said, "I'm tired of feeling like crap, I'd rather be dead. I refuse to go through the rest of my life feeling like this." "Oh, my God," I responded, "Not, I'd rather be dead. Didn't I ask you before not to talk or think so negatively because you block your healing and blessing talking and thinking like that?" I was taken aback since he appeared to have had a pretty goodnight's sleep. He was like Dr. Jekyll and Mr. Hyde. I thought to myself, "Do we have to go backwards," I asked, "plus, we have had some marvelous days and nights recently. Let's keep it positive and keep moving forward. Love and happiness." He never wants to go to dialysis, but he said, "I quit" this time. He cried and insisted, "I made up my mind, no more life support, no more dialysis, and I'm not going anymore. I can't, I just can't do this anymore. It's killing me." "Okay," I said, "but you're dying, anyway, let you tell it, so what's the big deal."

For I know the thoughts that I think toward you, says the Lord, thoughts of peace and not of evil, to give you a future and a hope. Then you will call upon Me and go and pray to Me, and I will listen to you. And you will seek Me and find me when you search for Me with all your heart. Jeremiah 29:11-13

He was dead serious and sounding like he was ready to die. Before, I thought he was just sick and didn't want to deal with it, but this time, he sounded very final, as if he was not going to deal with it anymore, final answer. I didn't know what to say but I managed to say, "Okay, sugar lump, but if you stop dialysis, you will surely die. Is that what you really want? Are you ready to go, be with the Lord?" He replied, "Yes, I am, I'm ready to die." I felt a chill, I felt lightheaded, hair stood up on the back of my neck, my legs were weak, and I began to get very emotional, trying to hold back tears because I could not believe my ears, sick or well, I could not imagine life without Rick and I had grown accustomed to taking care of him. I knew he hated dialysis and I was convinced that he was never going to like it, but he had to do it until he couldn't do it anymore – he is saying "this is it, I'm ready to die" but I wasn't ready and obviously God wasn't ready. I did not know whether to laugh or cry, why did he want to stop dialysis when it was giving him life? I loved dialysis because it was our lifeline and that was the only reason he was still alive. It was one of Rick's down days, I suppose. I was used to it, but I didn't want to be used to it. He was just having a bad moment, not a bad day, it was still early, he still had the rest of the day ahead of him to change his attitude. He wasn't going until God was ready for him anyway. I explained to him that I just wasn't ready for him to die, that I didn't want him to leave me yet, and he was not going to play God. I don't think anyone likes being sick. The congested heart failures and frequent trips to the hospital by ambulance had taken its toll on me, his heart and his other organs were in jeopardy having to work overtime to compensate for his failing kidneys and being a diabetic with complications so I'm sure he was tired, but he couldn't give up. That was not an option. My trust was not in the doctors, but in the Lord, and so was Rick's life. God helps us with the sin in our lives by redeeming us, reconciling us, justifying us and sanctifying us. We need continuing sanctification and cleansing from all unrighteousness and sin. He has a purpose, plan and will for every single one of us. The sooner Rick realized this better.

Trust in him at all times, O people; pour out your heart before him; God is a refuge for us. Psalm 62:8

I had taken on the role of wife, but I was not married to Rick, not yet anyway. I was ready to run, exercise my girlfriend rights as opposed to playing the wifely role. Things just weren't working in my favor. It was evident he only had me, and I couldn't take lightly the fact that we had been together for so long and he always considered me, treated me, and called me his wife. He desperately wanted to get married, but my excuses were: I did not want to be wife number three; I was divorced and had no interest in remarrying; and I loved being single, independent, and home alone. "We are already living as husband and wife, honeybun," he said, "please marry me and stop saying, 'one day'. I do not want my kids to get anything. It's my way of protecting you, it's the least I can do for all you've done and continue to do for me because you sure can't get rid of me. I love you too much. Let me look out for you like you've looked out for me, sustain and secure you for when I'm gone." What could I say? Him admitting he did not want his children to get anything was music to my ears because they sure didn't deserve anything. I had not thought that far ahead, but "sustainability" was food for thought and important, if something happened to him, God forbid, because I was still too young to collect my retirement. "I do not want to talk about death and if we do then let's talk about your wishes and desires for when you do die, let's talk about it while you're able" I said, "we will continue to work through your fears of dying. I'm sorry that you are having a setback but thanks for always having my back and thinking of me even when you're so sick, that's one of the things I love about you, and you are so loving, kindhearted and giving. Marriage will fall into place, eventually, when the time is right, be patient." I realized that I was being a hypocrite living in sin, so I knew in the eyes of God I had to do the right thing one day and I always justified it by making excuses all the while knowing we would eventually get married, I just wasn't sure when and I wasn't in any rush especially after Rick's stroke. I would get married when I was ready. I just wanted him to become God strong. Everything changes when you're aware of Jesus but if you don't want Jesus/God in your life He won't force himself on you so ask not, receive not; ask and you shall receive.

Ask, and it will be given to you; seek, and you will find; knock, and it will be opened to you. For everyone who asks receives, and he who seeks finds, and to him who knocks it will be opened. Or what man is there among you who, if his son asks for bread, will give him a stone? Or if he asks for a fish, will he give him a serpent? If you then, being evil, know how to give good gifts to your children, how much more will your Father who is in heaven give good things to those who ask Him! Matthew 7:7-11

I knew Rick was sick, but it irritated me to see him lay round all day, doing nothing. He couldn't do much, but he had no desire to get out of the bed to at least get washed up and to eat breakfast. All he did was eat, drink and sleep. He wanted to do everything lying down. It was quite pitiful to watch. He wouldn't even get up to go to the bathroom anymore. He was not trying to make this easy at all. "Body in motion stays in motion, body in rest stays in rest." He would sarcastically respond when I asked him if he wanted to go into the living or dining rooms, "Did I ask you to take me anywhere?" I was on the verge of losing my religion. The God in me would not allow me to stay in that space. I snapped back, with the quickness, to my loving, patient and compassionate self.   The flesh was getting the best of me, so I decided to use my gift of gab for God's purpose, and not my own.

Do you have the gift of speaking? Then speak as though God himself were speaking through you. Do you have the gift of helping others? Do it with all the strength and energy that God supplies. Then everything you do will bring glory to God through Jesus Christ. All glory and power to him forever and ever! Amen. 1 Peter 4:11

Rick was practically begging me to be his full-time caregiver at this point and he promised to be the model patient if I would take care of him, mainly meaning, quit my job. "I don't know," I kept repeating, "I just don't know." I did not want to commit or start something I couldn't finish but how could I keep saying no? I also needed to start practicing what I preached. I had to accept the fact that he needed a fulltime caregiver and deep down inside my gut I knew that God had chosen me and although I did not want to go against God or close any doors that God opened I didn't want to close, I couldn't commit to being a full-time caregiver especially since caregiving was a lifetime commitment.   Rick was already too much for me to handle, dialysis, lifting him, dressing, shaving, washing, pushing him in his wheelchair and we were still using the big oxygen tanks.   He was constantly struggling with depression and his doctor was in the process of increasing the dosage of his antidepressant and that depressed me.   I did not want his medications increased, I wanted them reduced, decreased, I wanted him taking less, not more. Life sucked at this point because I had finally accomplished my lifelong dream of becoming an authoress, so I continued to write nonstop and before I knew it I was finalizing book numbers two, three, four and several other books followed, but there was no time to promote them. While I was on a roll, I was also stuck in a rut, but I did not allow Rick to stop me from doing motivational speaking, workshops and seminars. I had become a life coach and public speaker overnight. Everyone and everybody were coming to me for advice, counsel and appearances. I never lost hope, but Rick's health issues brought everything to a fast halt. Although Rick's health problems started long before meeting me and the way he ate when I met him, it was inevitable that he would have some serious health issues. There was no excuse for his bad eating habits. He had diabetes since he was 25 years old and at the age of 46 everything came tumbling down. For three plus years we worked diligently to save his kidneys, prolonging dialysis for as long as we could. I couldn't understand for the life of me why Rick would not take his dialysis treatments like he was supposed to. I would be exhausted with all the special preparations and the constant doctor appointments. There was never time for me, but it wasn't about me. However, in the back of my head, I was very concerned about my own health and lack of sleep because I was taking darn good care of Rick but not me so much. God was taking care of me, He was the caregiver's caregiver, thank God. I could not have done anything without Him.

Patient [and] endurance is what you need now, so that you will continue to do God's will. Then you will receive all that he has promised. Hebrews 10:36

Rick and I were as different as night and day, complete opposites. He was a creature of habit who planned everything, and he saw the world as it was. He was sweet and quiet, never raising his voice. Whereas, I saw the world as a great big classroom and thought that I could not only change the world but save it too. I am spontaneous and totally unpredictable, loud and wild. We were opposites, but soulmates and God was our rock.

In You, O LORD, I put my trust; let me never be put to shame. Deliver me in Your righteousness, and cause me to escape; incline Your ear to me, and save me. Be my strong refuge, to which I may resort continually; You have given the commandment to save me, for You are my rock and my fortress. Psalm 71:1-4

I was working long hours, making a lot of overtime to make ends meet for both of our households. It was costing me an arm and a leg maintaining both places. Therefore, I was afraid to quit my job, I really needed that income plus we were living in such economically uncertain times and once I became a fulltime caregiver we would only have one income which was Rick's disability that he hadn't even started receiving yet and with the reduced income there would come struggling and heavy financial hardship, and we had enough to contend with already. It was a hard decision to make because I did not want to be broke, unemployed and struggling while being responsible for another person's life and well-being. I also knew that I had to rise to the occasion because he was not just any old sick man, he was the love of my life. We had already dealt with catastrophe after catastrophe.

Rick just didn't seem to understand that I couldn't work and care for him too, I just couldn't, and I was tired of defending myself to him. I still had no help and I still had to take off from work to let certain specialists in. For example, I had to be there for the respiratory therapist to qualify him for the portable oxygen since his oxygen had dropped to 82. I had to also be there when he was being evaluated for a motorized wheelchair. One good thing, Rick had the bomb health insurance and thank God, Medicare covered all his end-stage renal disease/dialysis expenses once it kicked it. We did not pay anything out of pocket and there were kidney funds that assisted with other expenses: household, diet, prescriptions, etc.

I needed help and suggested Rick's baby daughter who worked in a nursing home ne considered as his permanent caregiver, but Rick said, "she has such a dry, and nonchalant attitude and personality. No matter how hard I try to get close to her or reach out to her, she remains withdrawn and distant, she has low-self-esteem and just doesn't appear to take anything seriously, she's sweet but not that compassionate, patient, or strong enough mentally to care for me." He dismissed that idea, with the quickness. In her defense, she was a single mother, and he could not afford to pay her a sustainable salary even on a part-time basis. All Rick had to do was go to dialysis, physical and occupational therapies like he was supposed to, and he'd be able to take care of himself. I did not want to give up my job or my life and I felt Rick was selfish to expect me to do so. Nor, did I want to be harsh or appear mean spirited, but I was not going to be forced to do something that I did not want to do, so I tried to remain calm rather than argumentative. I would just keep praying.

Pray without ceasing. 1 Thessalonians 5:17

After praying and seeking God's guidance, and thinking about it day in and day out—caregiving, quitting my job, moving, marriage, all of it, had my mind racing. I was praying that God would help me win this race with grace. It soon became apparent what I needed to do. Slowly, but surely, I began to have a new attitude. I had to admit that I truly loved Rick way too much to ignore how much he really needed me. Money wasn't everything, it just doesn't hurt to have. I had some money saved and royalties coming in from my first book. Rick had exhausted his savings and was considering transferring money from his retirement. In the meantime, I was happy that he was finally receiving his disability checks because I was helping him pay his bills as well as taking care of my household, so it was all work and no play for me, and I basically worked to keep from placing limitations on things I wanted to do. Although I had practically moved into his apartment I hadn't given up my house and I hadn't quit my job. I know I said, money wasn't everything, but I was having a problem giving up the big paychecks, bonuses every three months, health insurance, and Christmas bonuses. The job was too stressful so if I eliminated it from the equation and devoted all my time to Rick, maybe my life would be less stressful. I just had to keep the faith and believe that God would work it all out. I decided to remain still and not act on my emotions, not just yet. I had to let God do what He do. Peace be still.

Therefore we do not lose heart. Even though our outward man is perishing, yet the inward man is being renewed day by day. 2 Corinthians 4:16

Returning home one Saturday evening after Rick's dialysis treatment, we barely got through the front door when blood began shooting out of his arm through the bandages like a water hose, splattering blood everywhere, clear across the room. I had to think and move fast. I rushed his wheelchair into the bedroom and somehow, I was able to reach the tape

96

and gauzes which were in the closet and in a space where his wheelchair could not fit. Thank you, Lord for your miraculous interventions, I could literally feel my limbs stretching and me performing the impossible. I felt like I was playing Twister. God was working behind the scenes and was helping us get through another episode. It was a miracle and when we returned to dialysis two days later, the doctor, nurses and technicians after hearing about our bleeding ordeal were amazed that I could stop the bleeding and not have to take him to the emergency room. They were quite impressed and so were we. Rick was impressed too because I remained calm, so did he. At this point, there was a lot going on with Rick. My heart was beating fast, I just didn't panic. Before Rick, I was an alarmist. Glory be to God for saving the day again and again. At any rate, that was confirmation that I was the bomb nurse (something I always thought I couldn't be because I hate the smell and sight of blood, vomit and poop). I cannot help but to think what might have happened had he been home alone, he probably would have bled to death. After that episode, I would probably never leave him home alone ever again. He meant everything to me and I knew he was an accident waiting to happen. Life was forever changing and before I knew it, life had become more of a juggling act between Rick's home, my home, and work. It was getting more and more difficult to manage the three. Working as an office manager/legal assistant posed problems for me in my caregiving role since my boss acted as though his business was suffering whenever I called out, or left early and that irritated me. Thank God, I never allowed my job to stress me out—work was a necessary evil. On the flip side, if I put myself in my boss' position, he depended on me to open the office in the morning when he couldn't, so I had to be there and on time. Lawyers cared more about their pets than they cared about humans. Regardless, I needed to determine what was more important in my life, and it had nothing to do with my boss. I had to figure out what was in the best interest of Rick, me, and my job. It was all on me and my decision only. My boss was not someone who could be ignored and whenever I called out he was going to have a problem with it, be very vocal about it, and I had no control over Rick's emergencies or how often they were going to occur. What I did know was that I wanted to be more available and supportive. I felt guilty when I left Rick at home alone and I felt just as guilty when I called out or had an emergency with him. I couldn't be in both places at once so every morning we prayed before I left Rick at home alone that he would be safe until I returned and when I called out from work I prayed that my boss would understand when I took off for Rick, but he never really did. Leaving Rick home alone stressed me out more than not going to work or my boss. I could always get another job, I couldn't get another Rick.

And whatever you do in word or deed, do all in the name of the Lord Jesus, giving thanks to God the Father through Him. Colossians 3:17

Putting things in perspective, God was first, I was second, Rick was third and my job was fourth so with my job falling in fourth place made it a no-brainer. I crossed my job off the list of things to do. It was the God in me that made me finally want to do caregiving around the clock. Moving forward, he has his own place now and he still needs me. I was really worried about him when I left him at his apartment alone now. I didn't want him to die alone and I did not want to discover him that way. Besides, he did make me feel somewhat guilty when he said, "If you truly love me you wouldn't keep wasting precious time especially since we do not know how much time we have left together. Let's face it, the things I want to do most, I can no longer do, but at least you and I can be together, in love and happiness, that's all I want, that is my last will and testament. I'll be sick, but you have that 'angelic caregiving spirit,' you're all I need. You're the most unselfish person I know, and you'll eventually come around, I know you love me and I can see it in your eyes that you don't want to leave me, but you must go to work. It'll be okay, though, quit your job, we can live off my disability." "I wish I could quit my job and not experience any hardship," I said, "I would quit in a heartbeat. It's just easier said than done. Let me think about it. I'm leaning toward that, it's just that mean green that's got that hold on me." He replied, "Take all the time you need. I'm not going anywhere." "I just don't want to be resentful later," I said, "when I make up my mind there will be no turning back."

Love is patient and kind; love does not envy or boast; it is not arrogant or rude. It does not insist on its own way; it is not irritable or resentful. 1 Corinthians 13:4-5

He left a lot on my mind and I couldn't help but to think what would happen to Rick if something happened to me? I knew this would be a very long goodbye if I were to commit myself to caregiving therefore I had to make sure that this is what I really wanted to do and could handle so I was talking to myself in the mirror trying to figure it out. I was always going back and forth about this issue and I was still hesitant. God had to be trying to tell me something because repeatedly my bible flipped to the same scripture:

There is no greater love than to lay down one's life for one's friends. John 15:13

"Was I ready to give up my whole life for another," I thought, "I was not ready to give up my fabulous four story house with a loft, three bedrooms, four bathrooms, and an overlook from the dining room into the basement. I was not looking forward to living in a one-bedroom/one-bathroom apartment with folks walking on top of my head; 65 miles away from all my family and friends, quit my job, and give up my financial freedom, all my freedom, for that matter. I had some big authoress-preneur dreams and I would be confined and unable to promote and market my books, something I really wanted to do. I was in my 50's, and I wanted to be selfish and just do me. I had every excuse in the world. Was I or was I not willing to make these sacrifices for another human being? I was fine, I was healthy, I had a nice home, a good job, I was living pretty large and in charge, making good money, I really didn't need Rick so what the heck, should I do?" I questioned myself and tried to convince myself repeatedly that he was not my responsibility. I tried not to get in my feelings, but I couldn't help it and I loved him so much no matter what. It was a very emotional and difficult decision to make. I had to dig deep and I began to think about my purpose here on earth and I just couldn't turn my back on such a good friend. Rick had been miserable for a while now and he was too sick to carry anymore unnecessary baggage or burdens. I did not want him to feel rejected, displaced or alone any longer. My heart was heavy, real heavy. I began to put myself in Rick's position. I was daydreaming, "God puts everyone in your life for a reason and some for a season. Rick was here for a reason. It was no accident that he and I met; fell in love, him being sick, and me being faced with the dilemma of caring for him possibly for the rest of our lives. Could this be a part of God's plan and could I be passing up a 'Jesus Calling' opportunity? What would Jesus do?" I knew the answer to that and it wasn't that I hadn't asked myself that question before, but the God in me would not allow me to overlook it or make any more excuses. It's an amazing feeling when you can feel God working on the inside of you. Thank you, Lord, I feel a change of heart coming on. I began to embrace the feeling. I just knew this had to be a test, one of the biggest ones I would probably ever encounter and knowing my purpose is to worship The Creator, and God's purpose was not for us to leave this life, just to get us into heaven, but He intends to use us for his honor and glory–Jesus Christ –becoming your life and living on the inside of you. He predestined, predetermined, orders our steps with his awesome power of wisdom to conform us spiritually so we can represent Him. We were both a work-in-progress, but I could feel God was in the process of sanctifying me, my thinking, feelings, actions, behaviors, integrity, character, addictions—sanctifying me in every aspect of my life. I felt as though I was going through a transformation and cleansing process. What a wonderful world this would be if everyone would just let God have His way with them. I even stopped smoking cigarettes. God took that taste right out of my mouth with the help of my grandson JR who hid my cigarettes after a family gathering, and when I chastised him about touching my cigarettes in the first place he expressed that he didn't want me to die or lose another grandma since his other grandma had recently passed away from a heart attack (who was a non-smoker, so he felt if she died and wasn't a smoker, I was definitely going to die because I was a smoker). Bless his little heart. I stopped right then and there. I was so touched, and I absolutely adore this kid for loving me so much and I only smoked two cigarettes a day anyway when I got home from work, but my doctor said, "one cigarette could be one cigarette too many." It was good for me to stop, not only for my health but for Rick too because although he had had a stroke he didn't stop smoking until I stopped. Thank God. God is powerful, and God is love. It has been a very long goodbye and we do not see any end in sight, so all we can do is keep the faith and keep praying.

O give thanks unto the God of heaven: for his mercy [endureth] for ever. Psalm 136:26

Change of Heart

I eventually had a change of heart. My granny and aunty has always stressed missionary work, service, helping the elderly, children, blind, deaf, mentally challenged, poor, sick, shut-ins, helping those less fortunate than me, and witnessing to others. "Once, I commit, there is no turning back," I thought to myself, "I have to be stronger than ever to take on this caregiving challenge. Are you ready? Yes, no, maybe so, I don't know." I still wasn't totally sure, but I was able and willing to give it a try. I asked God to search my heart and show me if there was some underlying wickedness going on. God knows my heart, my willingness, and He knows what I'm capable of. I prayed that God would lead me to walk in the will of God. I was waiting on the Lord to engineer my circumstances and give me His counsel, I was waiting on Him to lead and I would walk with Him.

I must be willing to give whatever it takes to do good to others. This requires that I be willing to give until it hurts. Otherwise, there is no true love in me, and I bring injustice, not peace, to those around me. Mother Teresa

More and more, God was touching my heart and I was seriously leaning towards accepting this caregiving challenge, but I still had my reservations, and although I had been resisting it, I was now approaching it with caution. I honestly felt as though I had put my time in and made my mercy deposits buy obviously not. I always helped everyone in need but what better way to prove to God that I loved Him than to give up my career, writings, and overall life for another human being. I could feel the Holy Spirit moving inside me and I was really feeling different about taking care of Rick. I couldn't explain the feeling, but I knew I would have to put all I had into the care of giving. I gave my job 150 percent, so caregiving shouldn't be that tough once I devoted all my time to it. I continued to pray for God's will.

Learn to get in touch with the silence within yourself, and know that everything in life has purpose. There are no mistakes, no coincidences, all events are blessings given to us to learn from. Dr. Elisabeth Kubler-Ross

God had placed Rick in my life for a purpose, so I had to do what I was called to do. I was beginning to feel honored that God had chosen me, He entrusted Rick's life into my care, and I wanted to make God proud and be the best darn caregiver that I could be.

I thank Christ Jesus our Lord, who has given me strength, that he considered me faithful, appointing me to his service. 1 Timothy 1:12

I was hit by the Holy Spirit. At first, I wasn't the least bit interested in taking care of Rick or even entertaining the thought. Before I was filled with excuses but now I couldn't see it any other way. The only explanation I have for my change of heart is that time heals everything and anything's possible with God's good grace. Rick deserved better. He feared dying and dying alone. That was fine, he can have fears, and he just can't give up. He will overcome the fears but if he gives up, he'll never know how much he could endure. Little did he or anyone know, I was also scared of him dying. My mind was racing with the thought, "love cast out fear and fear cast out love." It was stuck in my head.

What in the world does that mean? It seems that fear was getting in the way of love, but love was my direction and fear wanted to be my direction. That was nothing but God. It took me a while, but I chose love to be my counsel and I thank God for another miraculous intervention. Also, I knew I could always count on God, to be the caregiver's caregiver and take care of me.

We need to teach the next generation of children from day one that they are responsible for their lives. Mankind's greatest gift, also its greatest curse, is that we have free choice. We can make our choices built from love or from fear. Dr. Elisabeth Kubler-Ross

Moving forward, with a change of heart, I began to focus more on love and God. I started to see Rick not as a burden, not someone I didn't want to be responsible for or bothered with anymore, but instead I saw him as a priceless gift, a precious life that meant the world to me. He didn't deserve to be alone or rejected by anyone at this stage of his life. I also felt sorry for him because he was not getting the support he needed from either of his three children or family either, after all these years of being sick. It was painful to watch because he really needed peace of mind and a joyful heart.

Now the Lord of peace himself give you peace always by all means. The Lord be with you all. 2 Thessalonians 3:16

My kids, grandkids, and me were his only support system. His life was valuable, and he was an exquisite and honorable human being that really meant the world to my family too, and he meant way more than money and my job. Money isn't everything and it cannot buy health, love, happiness or life. I may not be able to save his life but if nothing else I could provide comfort, encouragement, nutrition and TLC.

Friends should comfort each other.

In that spirit, I recalled a bonding session between my mom and I on her deathbed, one that I will never forget, "Everything we have belongs to God," she said, "bank accounts, paycheck, furniture, houses, cars, and you are to manage it according to His glory, everything, I mean, everything is God's and He expects a return on the resources he entrusts to us. We are whole life stewards of our time, talent, testimony, treasure, and stewards are to be trustworthy. You are a steward by nature so never lose sight of the gifts God has given you. A steward doesn't own anything. You cannot take anything with you. Keep touching the lives of others in a positive way, keep following the way-maker's path and God will continue to bless and favor you. Service, keep doing God's work, you're on the right track." It was like my mother was right there beside me talking to me. She was a very intuitive, spiritual, intelligent, classy lady who read the bible faithfully and knew it from cover to cover. I could feel her presence. That was it! I don't know what took me so long, but I was finally ready to accept my life as it was.

And my God will supply all your needs according to his riches in glory in Christ Jesus. Philippians 4:19

My life was not complete without Rick so in sickness and in health I was ready to go all the way, I was even ready to get married, finally, and after all these years of being together, all Rick said when I finally said yes to marrying him was, "It's about darn time." "Well, you said, and I quote, "Take all the time you need," and you never tell a woman that." He replied, "That's a record by Roy Ayers, you did not have to take me, literally." We laughed and kissed! I confessed, "I am finally up for the challenge." The both of us broke into a duet, "Are You Ready" (by Barbara Mason). "Yes, I'm

106

ready, are you ready, yes, I'm ready, to fall in love, to fall in love, right now?" He was ecstatic, and I was happy to see him so happy. I felt good about my decision, but I honestly already felt like his wife anyway because that's how he always referred to me. It was just important to him to make it legal, make it right, and get that piece of paper. Rick was that kind of guy, my very own mister good bar.

Walk willingly at whatever you do, as though you were working for the Lord rather than for people. Remember that the Lord will give you an inheritance as your reward, and that the Master you are serving is Christ. Colossians 3:23

By the grace of God, I had finally made up my mind. What part of Rick needed around the clock care and supervision, did I not understand? Although I used to leave Rick's food in the bedroom I would often come home to a disaster, he had knocked over everything, all the time, plus I had even found him passed out, in distress, lying on the floor. No telling how long he had even been there. One occasion, he forgot to eat; another day he couldn't remember if he ate or not; items that belonged in the refrigerator were in the cabinet and items that were supposed to be in the cabinet were found in the refrigerator. He would put the bleach top on top of the dish liquid and the bleach would be found without any top. I couldn't understand why he was touching the bleach in the first place, since the dish liquid already had bleach in it. He was having incident after incident and he was a serious accident waiting to happen, a fall here and there, and I was afraid that one day I was going to come home, and he would be seriously injured or dead, it was a terrifying thought. It was no picnic lifting a dead weight grown man off the floor. I had also vowed not to ever leave him home alone a long time ago, so it was only a matter of time I'd live to regret it. I let my conscience be my guide, followed my heart and finally made the decision to quit my job, move to Virginia and take care of Rick fulltime. Since things were getting scary real fast I went to work the very next day and gave my boss a memo and he was really impressed with the memo and my decision to quit my job to take on such a huge responsibility. He wished me the best and we had the best couple of weeks working together that we had ever had in all the years we had worked together. So, I basically went from being a legal assistant to becoming a fulltime caregiver, just like that, overnight my title and life had changed. Yesterday, I was a legal assistant and today, I am a caregiver. It was official. I am Rick's fulltime caregiver. Finally! "Lord, give me patience, strength and endurance to be the best darn caregiver I can possibly be," I prayed. Rick was happy that I decided to be his caregiver, but he was still complaining about dialysis. He was overtaken by bitterness and anger.

Do not be overcome by evil, but overcome evil with good. Romans 12:21

Rick was beside himself. He was happy with my decision to finally give him the care of giving that he needed. He was such a sweetheart. He loved jewelry. I wasn't into jewelry because I have eczema but that didn't stop him from giving me a ruby birthstone ring for my birthday five months after we met and a diamond wedding band for Christmas the first year we were together. He really wanted to get married now. I always knew that Rick and I would get married but there was no need to rush it. We loved each other, and I knew that love would prevail and by the grace of God we will get through this together, one day at a time.

Seek the Lord and his strength; seek his presence continually! 1 Chronicles 16:11

A year later May 12th, Rick and I were finally married in a very small and private ceremony, right in our living room in the apartment in Virginia. My daughter and the clergy were the only other two people in attendance. It was sweet and intimate. It was the best day of my life, very romantic. Rick and I had a blast. He hummed and song all day long, "You Are My Greatest Inspiration" by Teddy Pendergrass. We had been together for over a decade and we were going through a lot more now than ever and I had to give him the type of security he needed, desired and deserved. We were already seriously committed to each other and married in our eyesight. God was blessing us despite our living arrangement, and moving forward we needed the goodness of God's light to constantly shine in our lives. We did not want to block any of our blessings or blessons by continuing to live in sin. Basically, we had to decide between good and bad, sin and evil. We wanted salvation and eternal life. We were deeply in love, so I couldn't say "no" to him about anything anymore. We had grown too close and been through too much. He loved me, and I absolutely loved and adored him and we both felt that we would be together until the end anyway. This does not mean that he did not piss me off from time to time but Rick and I were happy to finally be married and he loved having his own wife, it made him feel safe and secure. He really did love and appreciate me.

Therefore what God has joined together, let no one separate. Mark 10:9

I did the godly thing and I felt good about it. I had to do God's will. I am glad that I made the choice that I did when I did. Rick said it felt good to have his own wife. I was also happy to have my own husband as well. Our life was based on love, one love. Rick felt secure that I would not ever leave him now. He hadn't changed—he would still rather die than do dialysis. He was such a big baby, Baby Huey. I was like "Man, please, even AIDS isn't a death sentence anymore so get a life and stop complaining about dialysis. It is depressing the heck out of you, it's your lifeline and your last chance at life and no one can offer you what God offers you. He gives life to you every day. Show some love and appreciation to God for not snatching you during the night. Be strong, you need the will to live!"

But I will keep on hoping for you to help me. I will pray you more and more. Psalm 71:14

I felt helpless watching him slowly deteriorate, losing interest in reading especially since he used to be an avid reader. He was losing the little independence he had. He had no desire to do anything except stay in bed all day and night. He was my companion, my lover, my friend, my man, and we were road dawgs. He loved the outdoors, beaches, and exploring islands in the U.S., mountains, waterfalls, overlooks, panoramic views and picturesque sceneries. He loved holding hands, driving, traveling, short walks, picnics, bicycling, shopping, paddle boat riding, and paddle boarding. He loved doing whatever my little heart desired, so it was difficult watching him do nothing.

But because there is so much sexual immorality, each man should have his own wife, and each woman should have her own husband. 1 Corinthians 7:2

No matter what, I was devoted to him and I tried to keep him encouraged and inspired. It was nice having someone to share my life with that loved me so much. We loved cooking together and going out occasionally on date nights for seafood, veal or lamb. I cooked most of the time and Rick had a few darn good specialty dishes as well.

And now these three remain: faith, hope and love. But the greatest of these is love. 1 Corinthians 13:13

One day after dialysis, Rick and I went to one of our favorite restaurants, John's in Palm Springs for lunch when out of the blue, he said, "I do not know anyone who has as many things wrong with them as I do, and that's why it is so difficult for me to have as much faith as you. I'm always wondering, 'what's next?' If things are going well, I expect something bad to happen." I thought about what he just said and replied, "As a matter of fact, you are absolutely right, I don't know anyone either who has as many things wrong with them as you but if you keep expecting bad things to happen, nine times out of ten, bad things will happen." He continued, "I'm a stroke survivor,   insulin dependent diabetic with complications: I suffer with nerve damage and pain, high blood pressure, high cholesterol, anxiety, depression, constipation, right-side weakness (paralysis), glaucoma, wheelchair bound (non-weight bearing), bedridden, kidney failure, on dialysis thrice weekly, oxygen dependent and on 15 medicines, including prostate, reflux, nerve, antianxiety, anti-depression, heart, reflux, stool softener, blood thinner, pain meds, just to name a few – and let's not forget that I am the only man that we both know that has ever had a lump removed from his breast, his nipple detached and reattached. I also had a lump removed from my back. Not to mention, I need a damn kidney transplant, I just refuse to have one. I am a walking dead man." I commented, "Lord have mercy, OOG (Oh Our God) and on top of all that, let's not forget, congested heart failure, angina; vein, vascular and poor circulation issues, and 44 blood transfusions in one year, ouch, ouch, ouch!" He laughed, "Yeah, how did I forget about those 44 blood transfusions in one year? That's why I hate dialysis, it reminds me of having a blood transfusion." "Regardless," I said, "you are very much alive and blessed." "Sometimes, I feel blessed and cursed," he replied. You are stronger than you think, you've been through so much. May God continue to bless you.

See, I am setting before you today a blessing and a curse. Deuteronomy 11:26

"I am tired of suffering and living like this." Rick continued. I replied, "Whether you feel blessed or not, you are blessed to be alive and you better recognize. It hurts just thinking about all you've been through, and are going through, and that you may continue to go through, but what I want you to realize is, you are a true survivor, you are still alive, very much alive, a blessing, and my hero. You are blessed to have more things wrong with you than anyone we know so that makes you unique. It is bitter sweet. You have been through a lot but you're still here to testify. You were on 32, then 22 and now 15 meds, so that's a lot of progress, and we'll keep working on taking less and less. Like I said, you are way stronger than you realize or give yourself credit for. Meditate on healing and I promise you, God will help you. Ask not, receive not, and ask Him to shine some light in your life. God sometime uses us to answer our own prayers through His miraculous interventions. I can only do but so much—God already knows your needs, so talk to Him about your problems and pray without ceasing. Talk to him like you would talk to your father. Pray about everything.

Don't worry about anything; instead, pray about everything. Tell God what you need, and thank him for all he has done. Then you will experience God's peace, which exceeds anything we can understand. His peace will guard your hearts and minds as you live in Christ Jesus. Philippians 4:6-7

I knew that God could change Rick's mind because he sure changed mine about being his fulltime caregiver, giving up my house, quitting my job and moving 65 miles away. I sure wished that I could pray his darkness and sickness away. I prayed that God would shed some light in our lives.

This then is the message which we have heard of him, and declare unto you, that God is light, and in him is no darkness at all. 1 John 1:5

I did not want to dwell on the fact that he was the sickest person that I knew or have ever known. I'll say it again, "the one the sickest doesn't always go the quickest." I also blamed a lot on the pharmaceutical drugs' side effects since he was on so many of them for so long, and no medication is without side effects. I could see him wanting to do less and less and sleeping more which I didn't think was even possible. The dialysis treatments zapped all his energy and he was just tired of being sick all the time and having no quality of life. I couldn't blame him, and I just wanted him to be at peace and as happy as could be expected under the circumstances. I think he had reached his load limit. If you can only handle a little, God won't give you too much.

Use God's power to live a godly life and developing an intimate relationship with Him, simply follow His lead and Jesus' direction.

Rick was still holding his own and whether he liked dialysis or not he always looked forward to driving there and back three days a week since he had to go there anyway. However, one day on our way home he misjudged while turning left and was headed into ongoing traffic had I not grabbed the steering wheel. Although he was only driving for a short distance (less than a quarter mile) and a straight shot from where we lived, it had become too dangerous for him to continue driving. The ability to drive was the highlight of his life, and the one thing that added the most quality to his life, so when I told him he could no longer drive he was totally bummed, but he agreed that he would stop driving for the sake of his and others safety. After that we hired a driver to drop him off and pick him up from dialysis. It was easier for a male to lift him than for me to keep lifting him anyway. I was exhausted, totally burnt out. I was also wrong about caregiving—it was way harder than a nine to five. While he was at dialysis, I had time to write, exercise, work around the house and cook without any interruptions. Having a break four hours three day a week allowed me to get out more. My walks were quite adventurous and eventful, running into a bear one day, and a woodchuck, on another. When the Gaming Commissioner came he showed me an entire family of bears that lived across from my complex. My neighbors wanted to know what I was smoking. Well, the joke's on them. It was hard to believe that my besties, Angie and Brian Speddens did not believe my bear encounter. I gave them a pass because without hesitation, they would stop whatever they were doing to come to our aid or rescue. The Speddens were a Godsend, gifts from God. They were a lot of fun, loved to be threatened with a good time. Rick switched dialysis days to Tuesday, Thursday and Saturday so that they could help me with him on Saturdays. I would spend every Saturday with them after we dropped Rick off at dialysis. We went grocery shopping, ran errands, completed chores around the house and returned to pick Rick up from dialysis four hours later. Sometimes we went out to brunch or lunch. They even took me mud bogging, and to hit a tree with a bat to release frustration. It worked and was a lot of fun and just what the doctor ordered. If there was ever anyone in our lives that did way to much, it was Angie and Brian Spedden.

Let each of you look out not only for his own interests, but also for the interests of others. Philippians 2:4

They just could not do enough for us and they made sure that I was okay and had at least one good day out of the week and I always had the best time ever with them. I frequented their apartment when Rick was sleeping. They were a lifesaver! They partied every Friday night until 2:00 pm Sunday afternoon. Angie had to get ready for work on Monday so she cut the partying short on Sunday's. I called their apartment "The Downstairs Bar." It was the spot, the hangout. Even when my family visited me, we always went to the Speddens to get our party started. They were hilarious. They were my support system, party, family, friend, protector, getaway and lifeline. They were the best neighbors ever. Angie is a nurse, so she gave me a sense of security knowing she was right downstairs and worked right around the corner from the hospital we frequented. The entire Spedden family looked out for Ms. Jean and Mr. Rick and there are no words for our love and appreciation. Rick had a serious crush on our neighbor Ms. Linda who looked like Wonder Woman, and we both had a good friendship with her husband, Mr. Bobby. They loved talking sports and about Baltimore where Mr. Bobby was from and Rick had lots of family. Everybody was Ms. and Mr. I think it was out of respect for Rick and me because we were the oldest. Ms. Linda loved to share her great meals with Rick and I and she made the bomb frozen mixed drinks for me on the weekend and holidays. God had surrounded us with all the right people who genuinely loved and cared about us. Our neighbors were all phenomenal and helped us.

Happiness doesn't result from what we get, but from what we give. Dr. Ben Carson

Rick said he was sick and tired of being sick and tired of suffering. I thought we were passed this stage, but he was back to giving up so here we go again. How was I ever going to convince him to believe in miracles and in God's goodness and promises? After all these years, he still hadn't learned that Jesus is the key to life. He needed Jesus and he needed Him bad.

Jesus said unto Him, I am the way, and the truth, and the life. No one comes to the Father except through me. John 14:6

"There may not be much you can do about your many illnesses," I said, "but you can do a lot about your soul—and renewing your spirit."

116

A final word: Be strong in the Lord and in his mighty power. Put on all of God's armor so that you will be able to stand firm against all strategies of the devil. Stand your ground, putting on the belt of truth and the body of armor of God's righteousness. For shoes, put on the peace that comes from the Good News so that you will be fully prepared. In addition to all of these, hold up the shield of faith to stop the fiery arrows of the devil. Put on salvation as your helmet, and take the sword of the Spirit, which is the word of God. Pray in the Spirit at all times and on every occasion. Stay alert and be persistent in your prayers for all believers everywhere. Finally, be strong in the Lord and in the strength of his might. Ephesians 6:10-11, 14-18

God wants you to come to Him to find rest for your soul. He invites us to be still before Him, be quiet so we can hear His voice and set our hearts and minds at peace. I was totally relying on God to guide me, give me the strength and the words to say to Rick. I had to keep God first in my life and a part of everything that I did. I tried to make Rick understand that when you have God in your life you long for nothing, but love, joy, honesty, peace, harmony, trust and more God. I just wanted him to make this stumbling block a pleasant experience, not a lifestyle and especially not allow it to harden his heart.

Make the heart of this people dull, and their ears heavy, and shut their eyes; lest they see with their eyes, and hear with their ears, and understand with their heart, and return and be healed. Isaiah 6:10

I exclaimed to him, "there will always be hurt, pain, suffering, hardships and struggles, it is all a part of life and it makes us who we are.   When you comprehend and understand the love of Jesus you will be filled with all of God and his love crowding out your enemies, troubles, sins and sicknesses. You will begin to appreciate what is reality and what isn't. You have not fulfilled your purpose and it is hard to explain how we realize what God's purpose is for us since it will either be revealed or presented to us in the form of an unquestionable revelation, an opportunity, or it will be due to our journey or walk in life which builds faith, courage and strength in a more consistent way, a course that will also cleanse us and release us from our old ways of doing things and how we relate to life so we can begin to see and feel different spiritually. There is no special system or spiritual training required to determining what God's purpose is for us. Simply wanting to live a life that is filled with God's love is all you really need to start the process of spiritual reality. Also, the bible is the roadmap to faith and being a Christian, so every day we should pray, read the bible, be obedient, be grateful, be forgiving, exercise godly behavior, be gracious and witness to others.   The harmony of fulfilling your purpose will bring peace, joy, gratitude and blessings to all that you encounter. God's special gift to us all is that we be blessed and that we bless others—God is love."

Fix your thoughts on what is true and honorable and right. Think about things that are pure and lovely and admirable. Think about things that are excellent and worthy of praise. Philippians 4:8

Chapter 3

Stepping Out on Faith

Faith is an action. It is a clinging and a holding. Faith is what gives you hope to cope. When I was a young (teen) mom, my mother told me, that "clinging to hope and having faith is all you have sometimes, and something that never ends, never lose faith and you will always have hope, strength, and the ability to cope. It's all about the Holy Spirit, when you get older, you'll understand." I am older now, I understand, and I am happy for that blesson because I was tired all the time, frustrated, burnt out, overwhelmed and there was nothing I could do about it, so I spent much of my time hiding my feelings from everyone, crying in the shower, and praying overtime. I prayed a lot throughout the day. Emotionally, I was a wreck, but everyone thought I was strong. I was weak, emotionally, mentally and physically. I was drained. I was all he had so I had to hold him together. Amid everything else going on, all our helpers were leaving us.

Let us hold fast the confession of our hope without wavering for He who promised is faithful. Hebrews 10:23

Approximately five years into Rick's sickness, my sweet dear helpful earth angels and neighbors, Angie and Brian were moving from our apartment complex into a house not too far away, but far enough considering they would no longer be living downstairs and that was extremely disheartening. Rick and I knew that it was selfish on our

119

part, but we were devastated. It was always something changing in our lives, so I had become adaptable to change, but they were my framily, escape, getaway, break, and they also wheeled Rick outback for cookouts and family gatherings, so I wasn't excited about them moving at all. They also came upstairs to visit with us, and sit out front with Rick. My oldest son, Toby who often visited and who also helped us out had already moved 2500 miles away. Rick and I both were missing him and his family as it was. I wasn't sure this time we were going to be as adaptable to change. I had no idea what we were going to do since we relied on all of them for everything. They added balance and normalcy to our lives. They made things easier for us, and they were all a part of that village that kept us going. We had to figure out how we were going to move forward and survive without my son and neighbors. If there were a fire or if the wind blew too hard, Mr. Brian who was a gentle giant would be at our front door ready to rescue Rick in a heartbeat. Rick and I agreed that he didn't want them to move, like we had some real control over it. We thought about moving with them but that was totally unrealistic, unreasonable and unfair to them but, of course, they offered. They had been good to us and did more than enough for us, probably too much so it would be selfish to only think about ourselves, we had to take them into consideration and accept the fact that they were moving and there was nothing that we could do about it or to stop it. It is what it is!

Look not every man on his own things, but every man also on the things of others. Philippians 2:4

For all we knew, they could be moving to get away from us. I just bowed my head and prayed, "Lord, have mercy on us." We were genuinely happy for them, moving on up and into a house but we just didn't know what we were going to do without them. We didn't want to be a burden on anyone and not wanting them to move was purely selfish on our part – that was our problem – not theirs. They were our besties. Everyone needs an Angie and Brian in their lives, trust me, there is no one like them, best friends ever. We had just grown way too dependent on them for so much for so long and we were going to miss them and their angelic and generous ways. The Spedden's were genuine givers and we shared a deep friendship, more like family.

Love one another with brotherly affection.   Outdo one another in showing honor. Romans 12:10

With my son moving to California and the Spedden's move approaching Rick had a new assertiveness about him, an opinion, an interest, a voice, and a new attitude. I was loving it. He had come alive and was talking about moving to California. Not a day went by that he did not ask me a question about "California" and throughout the day he was very chatty about moving there. That was nothing but God! He was also talking about Toby and how much he missed him, his wife and the grandkids. It was all he knew and wanted to talk about. He wasn't talking about being sick, dialysis, or dying anymore. He wasn't complaining about anything, instead he had California on the brain and the Speddens' moving. He would talk about the pros of moving and there were no cons, he was 'rat to go.' I finally got a word in edge wise and asked him, "Are you serious, are you sure, you really want to move that far? Are you sure you don't want to go for a visit first, to see if we'll like it? Suppose we move there and hate it? There is no turning back once we buy a one-way ticket, give up this place, find a new place, start packing – but I haven't seen you this excited, interested or enthusiastic about anything for so long, so I say let's just do it, if you are serious, let's do it, let's step out on faith." I cried and prayed for God's guidance because I had no idea how I was going to pull this one off, travel 2500 miles from the east coast to the west coast, with a gravely ill husband.

Have I not commanded you? Be strong and courageous. Do not be frightened, and do not be dismayed, for the Lord your God is with you wherever you go. Joshua 2:9

He said, "With Jesus on our side, what can possibly go wrong? Nothing can be worse than here, it's like living in hell, and the weather alone during the winter is brutal. Sell the truck, let's go, I'm ready and thirsty for a change. I always wanted to go to California. We were supposed to rent a RV and drive cross country when we retire anyway. Plus, although I live close to my kids, they wouldn't have to treat me like I live thousands of miles away." I replied, "Well, we are early retirees now and we will just have to fly there because you are entirely too sick to drive or ride cross country. I don't expect the plane ride to be easy but at least it will be way faster than driving. If you are willing, I am too. I just need you to be patient, kind, and considerate of others as we fly. The airport could be crowded and congested." He promised to be a good boy. We laughed, and I was shocked when he said it again, "sell the forking truck, let's go, I'm 'rat to go' west. God bless my children. I can't wait to get far, far away from my kids." I interjected, "So you're running away from your kids, that's why you want to move to California?" He answered, "Why do I have to be running from something, why can't I be running to something?" "Excuse me," I said. Selling the truck was music to my ears and although he couldn't drive anymore his truck was still his pride and joy, his baby, he absolutely loved it and if he had someplace to go, he wanted to ride in his truck. I wouldn't think that he would ever part with it, and when he was willing to sell it, I knew he was dead serious and we were moving to California, final answer. He wanted out and we both needed a change. I didn't waste any time putting our plans into motion. I sold the truck with the quickness because I did not want him to change his mind. I started comparing moving quotes, found an extremely reasonable moving company, purchased airline tickets, packed, gave a lot away, he told his kids, and I told my two kids who still lived in the area. A few days before we were scheduled to leave, his baby sister stopped by bearing gifts of pajama pants, socks, underwear, shorts and T-shirts which was very generous, sweet and thoughtful of her. The day before our departure, my sister Cheryl gave us a going away gathering with family and friends in DC. Rick and I were extremely excited, and we could soon scratch California off our bucket list. On July 6th, my 58th birthday, my gravely ill husband and I stepped out on faith and boarded a plane to Desert Hot Springs (DHS), "California's Spa City" and is known for its naturally occurring water aquifers and home to the country's largest collection of hot mineral springs that contributes to the city's award-winning drinking water and the many boutique spas and resorts. It is beautifully situated between the San Bernardino National Forest, Joshua Tree National Park, and Mount Jacinto State Park, therefore offering lots of scenic views and outdoor recreation as well as the historical Native American history and culture, the Cabot's Pueblo Museum, displaying a variety of artifacts detailing a great and educational attraction for both the locals and tourists. Palm Springs, the President's playground and the celebrities' oasis and getaway, and the Cabazon shopping outlets are just a short drive from Desert Hot Springs as is easy access to San Diego and Los Angeles. We couldn't get there fast enough. We hadn't been this excited about anything for a very long time. God is so awesome! Thank you, Jesus! California, here we come!

Go home to your friends, and tell them what great things the Lord has done for you, and how He has had compassion on you. Mark 5:19

We were ready for a change that was long overdue. Bring it on—no more cold weather, snow, humidity or rain. We were moving to the best weather in the country and neither of us seemed to fear the threats of southern California's earthquakes and the desert heat. We made it to the airport in record time for the first leg of our flight. For the second leg, I had to run through the airport for about a mile and a half, pushing Rick in his wheelchair. We only had a 30-minute layover, hardly enough time to connect to the second flight, get something to eat, go to the restrooms which could be real tricky with a disabled husband. I had to take him into the ladies' room handicap stall with me, and God forbid if he had to use the bathroom on the plane or if he had an accident on himself, which he had never done before. When we finally arrived at the gate for the last leg of our flight, I was thankful, out of breath and we were the last passengers to board the plane rather than the first, like the first leg. In any event, we made it to our seats in time and was told that they were just about to page us. I ordered an Italian sub and wine, Rick ordered vegetarian vegetable soup with barley and a turkey sandwich. God, did it again! It was a long trip, a seven-and-a-half-hour flight and thank God there was only 2½ hours left on the second leg. Poor Rick complained the entire flight about his butt hurting and considering how long he had to sit on his butt, he was behaving quite well, no loud outbursts or whining. His jelly and sponge pillows weren't working but nothing could ruin my day or flight, so I held my hand under his butt massaging it for the entire flight, so he had no complaints at all. Overall, it was a good flight and a good trip. The main thing was we made it safely. It was a blessing we made it at all. When we touched down, we were happy to be on the ground and see my son and his family. We were overcome with emotion and peacefulness. We were feeling blessed. What a difference a day makes?

Grace to you and peace from God our Father and the Lord Jesus Christ. Philippians 1:2

Rick and I were anxious and excited to see our new home. Since we arrived in California on my birthday, my son and his wife gave me a birthday party that evening so we had to wait until the party was over to check out our new digs. We were exhausted from the flight and party, so we opted to wait until the next day. We were in Cali so there was no rush. It was going to be our home whether we liked it or not, this was home now, and we were looking forward to starting our new life in California. When the next day came, we could not believe our eyes, our new home totally blew us away, and it was a very nice two-bedroom house with great curb appeal. It was an adorable white house with a garage. We could fit our entire Virginia apartment into the living room alone of this house, we still had two large master bedrooms, plus a huge backyard about one-third the size of a football field, two olive trees in the front yard, sage on the side of the house; lemons, grapefruits, oranges, cacti and guava trees all around us, and the most amazing million-dollar mountain view; our street was off Mountain View. The tall mountains reminded me of Aspen, Colorado. We were smiling from ear to ear and could not believe our eyes. We were the happiest that we had been in quite a while, I mean really cheesing and smiling. We were going to have to stay with my son until the moving company arrived in another three days. We were so tickled we could have cared less. If Rick wasn't sick, we would have slept on the floor or even outside. Rick was more excited than ever and expressed to everyone how happy he was about living out whatever time he had left in beautiful and sunny California. He said if he died tonight he has lived a good life. We loved it. "We live in a paradise," he said, "I just can't believe this. I love you so much, I love it here. It feels like I'm dreaming, pinch me. The view is spectacular, breathtaking and I get to see it every day. This is just what we needed and what the doctor ordered. I said, "I love you so much." He said, "I love you more." I said, "I love you the most, and this is an amazing place and view. I feel so blessed and close to God here."

Rick smiled and said, "Me too, God is awesome, so powerful and mighty." "Yes, He is," I cosigned, "Praise Him."

We know that all things work together for the good of those who love God: those who are called according to His purpose. Roman 8:28

God did it again and again! Even if Rick got sicker and died, God forbid, we couldn't ask for much more than this because our lives had completely changed. "God will help us get through this ordeal," I reassured him, "and thank God, we stepped out on faith." It was hard to believe that we moved from opposite ends of the map, from one end of the country to the other, from the east coast to the west coast. It felt unreal. Being from Washington, DC this was a huge milestone in our lives and we were thrilled to take this journey together, during a very challenging time in our lives. He was happy and when he met his new team of doctors, he was even happier than I could have ever imagined. Praise God for keeping us and holding us together.

Two are better than one, because they have a good return for their labor: If either of them falls down, one can help the other up. But pity anyone who falls and has no one to help them up. Also, if two lie down together, they will keep warm. But how can one keep warm alone? Ecclesiastes 4:9

The doctors in California were all about having a quality of life and the doctors back east had basically given up on Rick because he didn't want a kidney transplant mainly because the recovery period was harder on the donor than the recipient and he was afraid that if my health was to decline he would not have anyone to care for him and he would feel responsible. Personally, I did not feel that Rick was strong enough for a kidney transplant although the doctors felt that he was an excellent candidate. The doctors felt that all his health problems were related to the diabetes and end stage renal disease (failing kidneys). California gave Rick more confidence and a new attitude about his health and living. It was a real pleasure to see him in good spirits and rejoicing despite after being sick for so many years.

Rejoice in the Lord always. Again I will say, rejoice! Philippians 4:4

The doctors were shocked to learn that Rick was not transported by a private medical plane from DC to California. We wish. That was funny though because they were serious. Rick was delighted when we went to the dialysis center. It was unlike any other dialysis center that he had ever been to before and we had been to many. One good thing about dialysis, there is a center anywhere we traveled. For the first time, we were at a center where I could stay with him in the treatment area during his entire treatment. There was no more dropping him off and picking him up later. I could leave him, but he wasn't going to want me to if I could stay with him. Also, his labs were so good that his treatment was reduced by 15 minutes. Fifteen minutes may not sound like much, but it was good for Rick since he was always asking to cut his treatment time short. Life was good. Rick was in a good mood and he loved having breakfast outside and sitting outside when the bugs weren't out because California's flies were irritating. My grandson (Nado) calls them ninja flies but other than the flies, we were living a wonderful and peaceful life. We were blessed to be on a staycation. Glory be to God!

The Lord bless you and keep you; the Lord make his face shine on you and be gracious to you; the Lord turn his face toward you and gave you peace. Numbers 6:24-26

Praise the Lord for his peace and comfort. Rick and I would say a prayer every day, a couple times a day. We were thankful but poor Rick was still praying for his children to have the opportunity to share this beautiful experience with him. Rick was always open-minded about the wrong things. If he did not see his children in Virginia, there was no way he was going to see them in California. I wanted to send him back to Virginia but, a phone call from his children would have sufficed. He did not want to go back. This was pathetic and such a critical time in his life when he really needed them. Rick tried blocking them out, but he remained troubled by his stepdaughter's attitude, treating him like he was already dead and refusing to pay him any rent at all, she stopped paying him before we left yet remained on his property. He said that she abandoned him when he needed her the most. We took an expensive move plus he told her repeatedly that he was on a special diet and had a bunch of prescriptions every month that his life depended on. Rick asked his son to get in touch with his sister, and his response was "that's between you and her, I don't have anything to do with you two's agreement" although he was the one who originally came to his father to say that his sister needed a place to stay. She never came to her stepfather; her brother came to him for her. Rick said his son could come to him for his sister, but he couldn't go to his sister for him, so he was crushed, and he was too through with him. He said he was sick and tired of his children showing him their ass to kiss. Rick, so graciously gave up his humble abode to his stepdaughter and her family. What an ingrate she turned out to be? It cut out our weekend trips. Rick still had the same phone number in California that he had in Virginia, so his children had no excuse for not reaching out to him. They refused to reach out to their sick father, what kind of children would do that? It was real hard for Rick to accept the fact that he was sick, and his children could have cared less.

Do not be deceived, God is not mocked; for whatever a man sows, that he will also reap. Galatians 6:7

His sister, his children's auntie also knew our contact information and landline number too. His children made him cry a lot and they made no attempt to get in touch with their terminally ill father. He was super hurt and baffled with his stepdaughter's disappearing act. She stopped paying rent, not for months, but for years. She purposely lost contact with her dying father to whom she owed rent. He was unable to get into contact with her because she changed her cell, home and work numbers. His children were a trip. He was also upset that his son who expressed an interest in buying the property in Virginia reneged on the deal and expected his sick father to pay the unpaid legal fees and expenses that he incurred when the deal fell through. His issue with his youngest child was just as bad, He purchased her a brand-new Yaris putting $6,000 cash down, making her car note just $249 a month and she let the snatch man take the car. Need I say more? He said, "These kids are going to be the death of me especially that stepchild of mine. Who would have ever thought that she would become a whole family of squatters? Who does that to their dying father though? She and her husband have to be mighty heartless to live rent free on a dying man. My son too, he knows how they're doing me too, and look how he did me, all I can see is asses to kiss." I felt bad for him. "Only if you let them, they cannot do any more to you than you allow them to do. Don't worry about them, pray about them, pray for them, and pray that they have a change of heart and be more loving and supportive because there is nothing you can do about them now and your freeloading daughter and her opportunist ass husband have every intention on living rent-free. You can evict them, but you are too sick for us to be bothered with putting someone out of somewhere they don't belong or have no right to be. I will not give any of your kids another second of my valuable time. You have done all you can do except evict her. Do not allow them to manipulate you, stomp on your heart or show you their ass to kiss anymore. Let it go and let God. One day, you may be dead and gone, but your stepdaughter and her husband too will regret squatting on you, and they will always need you before you need them." We agreed to get off that depressing subject and continued to make the best out of our new grand, stress-free, blissful, and lovely, spa staycation lifestyle. We felt blessed and we felt sorry for his children because they were grown, and it was too late to teach them manners, respect, responsibility and accountability but it was never too late to love or to cross the bridge of forgiveness. We prayed that their conscience and hearts would be touched, their souls lifted, and they have a change of heart toward their father before it was too late.

Be completely humble and gentle; be patient, bearing with one another in love. Make every effort to keep the unity of the Spirit through the bond of peace. Ephesians 4:2-3

Rick just couldn't figure out where he went wrong or what he ever did or did not do for them to treat him so badly when he was so gravely ill. No matter how hard he tried not to talk about his children, he couldn't help it and I couldn't blame him. He said that he couldn't get them out of his head, that it was just hard for him to accept that the fact that they had turned their backs on him the way they had. And, just when I thought we were finished with this conversation, he said, "I promise to haunt them for the rest of their lives and I will run my stepchild, step-son-in-law, step grandchildren and anybody related to them, it may even be more of them by then—I will run all their asses out of my damn house and off my property, you just mark my words, wait, you'll see. I don't know how but something's going to happen to run all of them out of there because she's a low down dirty snake in the grass. I would never have thought she would be the one to kick me when I was down, you just never know, do you?" He was shaking his head in disgust. What could I say? "Pray for them, I don't wish them any harm, you don't have too either, God will take care of them," I said. He replied, "Oh, I don't wish them any harm, but it won't be pleasant, karma is a you know what, that's all I'm saying so it will not be at the hands of me, it will be karma, what goes around comes around, and it won't be pretty. I might be dead and gone but it will happen," he said, "God will prepareth the table before me in the presence of my enemies. That squatter will get just what she and her family deserves." Personally, I had zero tolerance for anyone who mistreats or abuses another defenseless human being, no matter who it is but especially their sick parent. Rick's children wouldn't even call him to ask how he was doing. They were breaking his heart and they probably didn't even realize it. They ignored him repeatedly when he sent them at least two emails, so he eventually gave up on them altogether, and prayed that he could forget them the way they had forgotten him so long ago. All he wanted to hear was "I love you" and he wanted to tell them the same thing. He also wanted to extend an invite to Cali. I know he missed them although he acted as though he didn't. He was too compassionate a person not to be in his feelings about his children but less and less he talked about them. He felt all three of his children should be calling him, not him calling them. He and his son never made amends. Rick said, "I just want to forget about everything and everybody; forget about being sick and anything negative. Bottom line, if they don't want to be bothered with me, I sure don't want to be bothered with them. I just can't get them out of my head. I honestly do not understand them, I just cannot believe them. Forget those no good kids."

Discipline your children while there is hope. If you don't, you will ruin their lives. Proverbs 19:18

We were now living a life of staycation. It was a blessing, we would never have to worry about taking another vacation ever again, so his children were the last thing on my mind. We lived in a paradise, nine months out of the year; and it was hot as hell three months. Life was too good to be true. The heat was good for our bones during the real hot months which provided good natural vitamin D that we took advantage of 20 minutes or so a day. Rick and I were enjoying life to the fullest and he felt good most of the time. So much so we joked about going to the mountaintop to talk to God. That conversation went flat fast once we began talking about climbing up the mountain. We laughed as we envisioned me pushing his wheelchair up the mountain, snakes, getting lost, etc. So much for that. Dialysis was going well, his attitude, diet, weight, fluid control, labs, everything was good. I was always receiving complements at the dialysis center, doctors and hospital stays about my attentiveness, patience, how well-kept/groomed Rick was, how pleasant we always were, and how I never left his side. I checked into the hospital like most people would check into a hotel for weeks at a time, with my suitcase in hand. Everyone always had such glorifying things to say to us. I was flattered but I wasn't doing anything special. I was doing what I was supposed to do – God's will and taking good care of my husband like I was supposed to.

And now, Lord, You are God, and have promised this goodness to Your servant. 1 Chronicles 17:26

Rick was in a good mood and on his best behavior at dialysis today. On the way home, he said he couldn't wait to get home, sit out back and watch God's artwork in the sky, the clouds shaped like humans, animals and sea creatures. He even talked about getting into flying doves since we had so many visits our backyard, but I knew that was just talk. Rick was much happier and hopeful in California than he ever was back east and that was quite refreshing. He may not have been fine with having a stroke and being a sickly person, but he sure was enjoying his unemployment and freedom to sleep and do nothing. No matter how long it last, Rick was in a good place and it was great to see him happy for a change. I was hopeful.

May the God of hope fill you with all joy and peace in believing, so that by the power of the Holy Spirit you may abound in hope. Romans 15:13

Just when I thought Rick had it all together and was doing better, he decided to tip the scale of hope and cope. Rick was back to blaming God for his sickness. He was like most people, all about God when everything was going his way but when things weren't going so well, he was weak. I do not know how he expected God to help him if he was not willing to help himself. "Hold on to Jesus and Jesus will hold on to you and not let you go," I said, "life brings circumstances, misfortune and sometimes sickness, not God. God did not let you have a stroke. I reiterate, sometimes bad things happen to good people. We all have felt hopeless at one time or another and most of the time we do blame God because we believe He has the authority to keep bad things from happening to us but that's when God puts us to the test to see if our life is worth living or not, to see how we will respond, and how much faith we have, if any. His health problems were not going to go completely away so I am sure it was a horrible feeling of hopelessness for him therefore I am not trying to diminish his sickness, I just didn't want to be an enabler or cripple him any further. "When we live our life with faith in God," I said, "His eternal rewards are tremendous and no matter what we go through, God will help us get through it, but I really want you to understand that God had nothing to do with you having a stroke and God is moving in your life and you may be down, but you're not out." He agreed, "Nope, I'm not out, not yet."

Without faith it is impossible to please God because anyone who comes to Him must believe that He exists and that he rewards those who earnestly seek him. Hebrews 11:6

That was the spirit! I wanted him to see that God was rewarding us despite everything else that was going on in our lives. We thought this type of life and happiness was impossible for us especially after his stroke. Anything was possible and as far as I was concerned, things were much better than ever.

For nothing is impossible with God. Luke 1:37

God does work in mysterious ways. His timing, divine and miraculous interventions are always on time. God did it again and again and again! Rick had to see how God was moving in our lives, always making a way out of no way and he hadn't been in the hospital since he arrived in California. Praise the Lord, thank You, Jesus, Hallelujah!

Chapter 4

Dementia

After living in California for a little over a year, I became concerned when I noticed more and more impairments with Rick's memory, thought and communication abilities. At lunchtime, Rick was unable to recall what he ate for breakfast, or couldn't remember whether he had eaten at all, and that seemed to me to be more than just a senior moment. I immediately took him to the doctor who diagnosed him with dementia which causes problems with reasoning, remembering, thinking and behavior severe enough to interfere with one's daily routine. Diseases, injuries, and even nutritional deficiencies can cause dementia. In either case, dementia is caused by damage to brain cells which affects the way you think, feel and behave. Other causes of dementia include head trauma, Huntington's disease, Creutzfeldt-Jakob disease, and HIV. Dementia is a reference given to brain disorders which affect cognition, social skills, and memory with Alzheimer's being the most common form of dementia. Rick had the second most common form of dementia, vascular dementia which occurs when a stroke damages the blood vessels to the brain. Vascular dementia symptoms are like Alzheimer's except they come on suddenly. Rick got lost on our street, I found him and his wheelchair at the bottom of the street; he had difficulty speaking (often using wrong words, saying bizarre, unpleasant, inappropriate and strange things); shortly after eating, he had no recollection he had eaten; he thought a hospital I.D. bracelet on his arm was an arm band for re-entry into an amusement park; he sang into a knife for a microphone (holding the blade part in his hand); he was unable to remember basic personal information or understand new things; his personality and hygiene changed; he was combative, offensive, and frightening with his bizarre behavior (snatching, throwing things, name-calling, swearing, threatening, hitting, spitting); the ability to put more than one memory together, make an old memory a new one and unintentionally lie; put underwear on top of his head for a hat; making unreasonable requests; no longer recognized loved ones and mistaking them for others in his past.   He wasn't only confused, forgetful and unable to recognize family and friends, he began having difficulty following directions, being reasonable, he was more depressed and anxious than usual, repeating himself, difficulty holding his head up, and eventually he lost all mental capacity.   He would not talk, he would have screaming and yelling rampages, and fits of rage that would last for hours. I did not know whether to feel sorry for him, commit suicide or homicide. How I reacted or responded often determined his mood or attitude since he was experiencing a lot of personality changes, so I constantly reminded myself to remain calm, patient, and proceed with caution.

That your faith should not be in the wisdom of men but in the power of God. 1 Corinthians 2:5

Dementia patients could be dangerous. Rick would accuse me of not feeding him. At times, he did not know who or where he was, and he would scream, "police, police, help, help, police" to the top of his lungs until he got tired. He acted as though someone was holding him hostage or trying to kill him. What was on his mind? What was he thinking? It wasn't personal, so I had to maintain my patience despite the madness. I had to refrain from being angry at him for his bad behavior and language.

And "don't sin by letting anger control you. Don't let the sun go down while you are still angry." Ephesians 4:26

Dementia was making it very difficult to hook Rick up for his peritoneal dialysis treatment. The doctor prescribed some sublingual lorazepam since I literally had to drug him to give him his dialysis treatment these days. It is hard for you to remain calm and patient when someone is spitting or fighting you, so I had no choice. He wasn't talking to me. He didn't know me when he had these outbursts and fits of rage. He was talking to his sister, his first and second wives. Sunshine was his sister and I was both ex-wives, so I got a double-whammy. Dementia was hard and a whole other phase of caregiving that was close to impossible to endure. I was missing his smiles, hugs and kisses and I was totally exhausted. I was just as lost and confused as he was, but I had to remain in good spirits despite it all. I could be his eyes, ears, legs and arms but not his mind. Every time I tried to tell him that I was not his first, but third wife, he would go off, call me a liar and curse me out. That was hilarious. I thought if I played along with him and acted like I was his ex it might calm him down but that didn't work either, it just got worse. It all depended on his mood. I was damn if I do and damn if I don't. Obviously, he had a lot of unfinished business and a bunch to get off his chest or mind. He was resentful, belligerent, angry, nasty and hateful towards his first and second wives but the first wife, the mother of his children and the one with the stepdaughter, he was like a creature from the black lagoon towards her. He unleashed all his anger on her. I have never heard or seen Rick, or anyone act like that before. I felt bad that he was sick and getting that upset. It couldn't be healthy for him to behave this way. It wasn't even healthy for me to watch. I was frightened. His behavior and attitude were very ungodly and mean-spirited. I prayed. He looked so confused. My poor hubby.

Know this, my beloved brothers: let every person be quick to hear, slow to speak, slow to anger; for the anger of man does not produce the righteousness of God. James 1:19-20

He was recalling more and more events from his past, including dead people. It appeared that he had one foot in the grave and one foot out so if he were really on his deathbed I didn't want him to be in such bad spirits and feeling so much hatred because he may not get his wings, after all. You just never knew with Rick because he was deathly ill and while he did not have any quality of life, he always managed to spring back to a livable state of consciousness, and his heart was still ticking. I had to figure out how to refocus his mind and re-channel his energy. I didn't know what else to do except give it to the Lord and pray that Rick does the same.

For if we live, we live to the Lord, and if we die, we die to the Lord, so then, whether we live or whether we die, we are the Lord's. Romans 14:8

After all these years, I still feel like I'm fighting a losing battle and I was beginning to resent caregiving, something that I had always feared would happen. There are so many conditions (over 80 different types) under the dementia umbrella so learn the type and stage of dementia your loved one has so that you will know how to communicate with them, locate caregiver support groups, implement home safety tips; understand legal matters, manage behavioral problems, develop relaxation techniques, and seek information and support for in-home dementia caregivers in your state or county that provides educational materials, information and resources to assist caregivers caring for patients suffering from dementia. Dementia is a confined and intense level of caregiving, so you may need the help of a professional specifically trained or skilled to work with dementia or Alzheimer's patients.

Caregiving has taught me a lot about me, my heart, my faith, strengths, and most of all, how blessed I truly am. I am the voice of experience when it comes to caregiving because I provided round-the-clock intensive caregiving to my husband for seven years. I was also a caregiver to others however the challenges of coping with a dementia patient on dialysis was much more emotional, stressful and required more caregiving for many years. The challenges were much different than those faced by the average caregiving experience.

For we are God's masterpiece. He has created us anew in Christ Jesus, so we can do the good things he planned for us long ago. Ephesians 2:10

Peritoneal vs Hemodialysis

I wish I knew then what I know now about hemodialysis versus peritoneal dialysis and that Rick had started peritoneal dialysis a lot sooner. Peritoneal dialysis allowed us to dialyze at home for longer and every day, thus cleaning toxins from the body more regularly, like having a real kidney. That's exactly what dialysis is—an artificial kidney. The beauty of peritoneal dialysis was that he could do it as he slept and by doing it so often for so long prevented the body from building up hardly any toxins in the body, the diet was more flexible than hemodialysis, and gentler on the body. He literally hated hemodialysis at the center three days a week because it was too draining, zapped all his energy, very time-consuming (including the commute and treatment time), the diet was strict, totally inflexible, and extremely tough since he had to follow four diets: diabetic, stroke, heart and kidney-friendly diets combined into one. From time to time patients were rushed to the emergency room during or after dialysis treatment; he and other patients suffered from fluid overload and the center often removing too much fluid, serious drops or spikes in sugar and blood pressure to patients experiencing strokes or heart attacks. It wasn't easy at all. Nothing about Rick being sick was easy. End-stage renal disease is no joke so take care of your kidneys as well as your other vital organs. While Rick's diet was challenging and involved a lot of detail, it was doable, and I welcomed the challenge because I was a natural born foodie. The meal part gave us both something to look forward to that was very comforting and he knew his food was made with a lot of love and made especially for him. It was just time consuming and time was not something I had a lot of. With peritoneal dialysis, his meals did not have to be so methodically planned like hemodialysis. Rick was a thin man, but he has always had a great appetite before and after the stroke. Being such a thin man, thank God, he never lost his appetite.

The bible is a promise book and God is so awesome.

When one person is sick, the whole family is sick. California gave me everything, especially the tranquility with that breathtaking million-dollar mountain view which made me realize the power in having peace of mind. I had a great sense of comfort and control now. It was like God personally sent us to Cali. He sure made it possible and put the opportunity before us and I thank God that we took that leap of faith. When we went to Rick's new primary care doctor's office in California, we never waited like we did back east, we were seen right away. Rick's new doctor saw one patient at a time and he was very thorough. When we arrived at home that evening after our doctor's appointment there was a contraption at our front door, something I had only seen in the hospital. I was not sure what it was, but Rick identified it as a lift. Hallelujah, praise the Lord, thank you, Jesus. Finally, I was getting hospital equipment that I really needed for providing the best in-home caregiving that I could. The next day a physical therapist showed up to educate me on how to use the lift. He and the lift were a Godsend. We were being blessed with abundance. People at the dialysis center, church and neighbors were always giving us fruits from their trees.

And God will generously provide all you need. Then you will always have everything you need, and plenty left over to share with others. 2 Corinthians 9:8

Rick and I had come a long way, but we still had a long way to go. He was finally scheduled for surgery to place the dialysis catheter in his stomach for peritoneal dialysis, he had waited a long time to do dialysis at home. Back east we did not have the space to store all the medical supplies needed nor did they offer the peritoneal training at our dialysis center at that time. He was thrilled at the thought of never having to go to the hemodialysis center again except for lab work. Hemodialysis or peritoneal dialysis is not for everybody, but hemodialysis was very hard on Rick's body to the point it was killing him. He really liked the California dialysis center better than most, but nothing would be better than being able to do it at home, according to him. I believe in taking control of your own health, but I wasn't enthusiastic about his surgery because I didn't think that he was strong enough for any type of surgery, but he was determined, and he and the surgeon were ready to get it done and over with. No matter what I said, it was his body and he was having the surgery to place a catheter in his stomach. All I could do was pray, so I prayed for Rick, the surgeon, the anesthesiologist, and everyone else in the operating room. God knew how sick he was and how bad he wanted this surgery, so I left it in the Lord's hands.

But when Jesus heard this, He said, "It is not those who are healthy who need a physician, but those who are sick. Matthew 9:12

Rick had the surgery and came through it with flying colors. Praise the Lord! Unfortunately, the night of the surgery Rick bled into his stomach, and loss consciousness. He was persistent and insisted upon this darn surgery and I had reservations about it all along. I was just being supportive because I knew this was what he really wanted. Rick said either way he was going to die so he would take his chances and that's what he did. When I realized that his oxygen machine had stopped, it was a matter of life and death. I immediately called 9-1-1 and began CPR. It wasn't as bad as we thought, thank God. He was hospitalized and released a few days later and was able to do dialysis at home afterwards. We were used to setbacks and comebacks at this point. I would hook him up at bedtime and take him off in the morning. He would sleep through the entire treatment. He was doing well and feeling good about dialyzing as he slept. His diet was more flexible, and he loved it. He said he had died and gone to heaven. Although he hadn't been doing it that long, he was not having any of the side effects so far: upset stomach, headaches, coughing, peritonitis infection, chest pain, flu-like symptoms, elevated blood pressure and blood sugar. As a matter of fact, his blood pressure and sugar had never been better. Rick was happier now than he had ever been and so was I. We were living in the now. His memory was even renewed, just a little. We're just happy that he survived the surgery which he barely did if I hadn't noticed he wasn't breathing, he would be dead. Rick was real resilient, he always sprung right back. We always paid close attention to his potassium and phosphorous intake so that he would not get a buildup or overload in his body. People with working kidneys do not have to worry about that since working kidneys will automatically release the unwanted potassium and phosphorous from the body. I had to cook fresh meats for sandwiches – turkey, chicken and roast beef, he could not eat any processed foods, cured or organ meats and I would soak potatoes for four hours or overnight to get the potassium out before cooking them. Rick loved cheese and I allowed him a little white cheese and tomatoes in moderation. We had to switch from wheat bread to white bread. Life was forever changing so peritoneal dialysis offered a lot more flexibility and was a change Rick welcomed. Thank you, Jesus!

Do you not know that you are God's temple and that God's Spirit dwells in you? If anyone destroys God's temple, God will destroy him. For God's temple is holy, and you are that temple. 1 Corinthians 3:16-17

On top of everything else, Rick had a mild heart attack and had to have a stent procedure done and when he was assigned to his hospital room the nurse asked me, "How have you been treating his bedsore and how long has he had it?" I had no idea what the fork she was talking about. In puzzlement, "What bedsore," I asked, "he doesn't have a bedsore." I thought she was mistaken, she had to be. They were making me lose my religion. He has NEVER EVER had a forking bedsore, if he has one it's the hospital's fault, he's been sick for almost seven years and never had a bedsore," I cried. The doctor walked in and said, "Your husband is immobile, so a bedsore was inevitable. He has one now and there is no one to blame. It's probably been coming for a long time. Bedsores don't just happen suddenly, in a day or overnight." Rick replied semi-consciously, "Yeah, they did it, they put me on a steel operating table, no cushion or mattress, no bedding, nothing and that's what caused it to bust open like that." While I was speechless and shaking my head, the doctor ignored Rick's outburst, and leaned him over for me to see his behind and I could not believe the sore on his tailbone. It was an open wound. It still gives me the chills to think about it. I put my hands over my mouth in disbelief and I cried so hard that I was inconsolable. I boohooed like I had never boohooed in my life because I had been working too hard for too long trying to prevent a bedsore or any sores or ulcers for that matter, but he really didn't have any fat on his bones and being on dialysis we were always struggling with him to consume enough protein, so I had to accept that it comes with the territory, from all the laying and sitting. He loved the bed before he got sick and now he had an excuse not to get out of the bed. At home, I used lots of pillows to support the different positions and I moved him frequently, but he did complain the entire trip on the plane that his bottom hurt. Prior to that he never appeared to be having any butt pain. A few weeks later Rick was taken back to the hospital where they had to place a feeding tube through his nose because he refused to eat. This was getting scarier and scarier. His whole body was breaking down and things were changing and going downhill real fast. He wasn't talking much anymore. This was only his second time being admitted to the hospital and the second time he was like a corpse, and it was not my imagination. What were they giving him? What were they doing to him? Was I paranoid? This time I made an appointment to speak with the entire team of doctors in person, all together, I needed some answers; I wanted to know what was going on, what was happening to him?" I explained to the heart surgeon that no matter what, they should never have place him on a bare steel table knowing how thin and fragile his body was. I also learned that wasn't the first time. When he had his upper GI,

147

he said they did the same thing. What the heck is wrong with this hospital's procedures? There were a lot of doctors, nurse practitioners, nurses, physician assistants, specialists, respiratory therapist and the hospital administrator who started off by asking, "What can we do to make this right, what do you want us to do?" I was pleased with their approach. "You can start by healing that darn bedsore, with the quickness. I do not want it to turn to gangrene," I cried, "that's all I want you to do, just heal it, please." They all looked at me like I was crazy, like gangrene was a foreign word. The wound specialist responded, "we will assign you a wound team and the necessary supplies and medications, but we cannot make any guarantees because bedsores are very difficult to heal but we will do our best." I was totally discouraged and for the first time, I felt as though I was really about to lose him. He was falling apart at the seams, not eating, not talking, barely moving. After I left the meeting I went to his room. I thought he was asleep but out of nowhere, I guess the meds had finally worn off, he started swearing and screaming like a maniac. I wanted to shut him up, but I couldn't, and I also wanted to crawl into a hole and hide. I had to remind myself that I was a child of God and that he was a very sick man. His brain was not working right and as scary as that was, I had to be patient and strong. I could not control him, and he had no control over himself. I felt as though I was fighting a losing battle, again. He was losing his mind, slowly but surely, so I would have to learn some new techniques with dealing with this new and outrageous behavior.

Blessed [is] the man that walketh not in the counsel of the ungodly, nor standeth in the way of the sinners, or sitteth in the seat of the scornful. But his delight [is] in the law of the LORD; and in his law doth he meditate day and night. Psalm 1:1-2

Rick called me everything but the child of God. I thought I was all cried out, but I wasn't. I had been his everything and anything else that he wanted me to be. It was hysterical, rather hilarious, at first, and I was laughing but it went bad fast. All I had done for that man he had the nerve to disrespect and dog me out like that, I couldn't believe it. He was making me lose my religion. That wasn't anything but the devil. He was speaking very disrespectfully saying horrible things, name calling and yelling to the top of his lungs for the entire hospital to hear him. In between cursing, he said he wanted to die and was begging, "Let me go," he yelled, "let me go, please let me go. I want to die, let me go." I told him it wasn't up to me. He told me to "shut the fork up," ain't nobody talking to your no good ass. Get out of my damn face. I hate you, and I'm sorry I had any kids with you." I was laughing hysterically to keep from crying and cussing him back until I realized he wasn't talking to or about me because he and I did not have any kids together. Hallelujah! I was a little relieved that he was not talking to me instead he was talking to and about one of his execs because those ugly words were coming from a man who always told me how beautiful, godly and great I was, but he sounded like he hated the person who he was talking to. Although he wasn't talking to me, I still had to leave the room because he was being brutally mean and loud. I was crying uncontrollably now, the tears kept flowing. I honestly did not know how to process what had just happened. As I walked down the hall confused and sobbing, a nurse and two doctors ran behind me to tell me not to cry or leave because he wasn't in his right mind and that he wasn't talking to me, it was the disease. I told them, "I know he wasn't talking to me, but it was horrible to see him this way, out of control, so cantankerous, and the fact that the doctors couldn't do anything to help him made me realize he was way further gone than I could have ever imagined. If y'all can't help him, how am I going to be able to care for him now?" I asked. He was cussing his first wife out like a sailor. I have never seen him act or speak like that before. Rick used to be the quietest and sweetest man you could ever meet. Wow! It is always something. I'm shocked. Help us, Lord, we may need a little extra, so give me strength to endure this phase of our lives."

He giveth power to the faint; and to them that have no might he increaseth strength. Isaiah 40:29

In any event, I was totally embarrassed, and it was weird how he was looking through me, starring me down but talking and addressing someone in his past. He would never act like that especially on the heart unit, if he were in his right mind, he was always such a gentleman and considerate of others, but this monster didn't care; he was so mad and angry, and I had never seen this explosive side of him before, so I just prayed that he would stop screaming and cussing for the other patients' sake. I sure couldn't calm him down and it appeared that he wasn't aware of what he was doing or saying. He was a crazy wild madman. One of the staff physicians led me back to a conference room and explained to me that Rick had dementia. I felt bad for him because on top of everything else he was losing his darn mind. This was one time that I was glad he was in the hospital. He obviously was getting worse. "Give me patience and strength, Jesus," I cried, "let me be thankful for all things, good and bad. It's life, just a hard life! Have mercy on us, Lord!"

The LORD is gracious, and full of compassion; slow to anger, and of great mercy. Psalm 145:8

HELP!

I finally arrived home from the hospital and was looking forward to taking advantage of some "me" time while he was at the hospital. I needed to pull myself together, I had a little time to reenergize. I sure needed too. Again, dementia patients required way more training than routine caregiving, they required a skilled nurse with a specialty in dementia and Alzheimer's. "How do I proceed from here, I require your guidance, Lord. I'm not saying I can't, I'm saying I do not know how to take care of a dementia patient. HELP!"

I will lift up my eyes to the hills—from whence comes my help? My help comes from the Lord, who made heaven and earth. Psalm 121:1-8

I needed to focus on me and my health for a moment. I was feeling overwhelmed and speechless about what I was going through with Rick. I was losing my spirit and joy. I was close to collapsing myself. One thing for sure, God would continue to help Rick with his spiritual body. I am nothing without Them, so I put all my trust and faith in Jesus and my Heavenly Father.

It is sown a natural body; it is raised a spiritual body. If there is a natural body, there is also a spiritual body. 1 Corinthians 15:44

I poured a glass of Pinot Noir. Cooking always relaxed me so I looked forward to preparing me a nice meal. I was gleefully singing and dancing around the house, glad to finally get a break so I was going to take advantage of it. The phone rang, and I started not to answer it because I had been home for less than an hour, I really didn't want to be bothered with anyone, but it was a good thing that I answered the phone because it was the hospital calling to say that they were discharging him, and I needed to pick him up ASAP. "OOG (Oh Our God)," I said, "Now, really, right now, I'm sorry, what do you mean you're releasing him right now, that's ridiculous? You can do more for him there than I can do for him here. I do not have a problem with him coming home–I just cannot transport him. He requires ambulatory transport." The nurse replied, "He should arrive within two to three hours, at our expense." "Thank you," I cried, "thank you. Goodbye." I hung up, in total shock. Shaking my head, I thought to myself, "What the heck?" He was coming home – so much for me eating, relaxing and reenergizing myself. I never got to put my salmon, potato, radishes, brussels sprouts, and fried artichokes with crabmeat dip. I was pissed! No matter what I did, I just couldn't catch a break. I had to start cleaning his room from top to bottom. Poor Rick, deep down inside, he probably felt unwanted and unloved. He just couldn't process it all. I began to cry and pray, "Oh God, please help me to comfort him, give me the strength Lord to take care of him the way he needs to be cared for. Give me the care of giving spirit and power to comfort my husband and bring him to his salvation." We had twin hospital beds in our bedroom, one for him and one for me. One was electric given to me by a very nice wound care specialist who worked at the hospital and the other one was covered under his medical insurance. I cleaned our room like a mad, mad housewife and I was done in no time, but I still needed to shower, eat, power nap and I was running out of time and steam, I was losing energy fast, but I was always tired. I continued to listen to some instrumental-only music which relaxed and stimulated my body and mind. It was looking bad for Rick and I was just as afraid of losing him as he was of dying. I prayed for victory over fear.

Yes, I will help you. Isaiah 40:10

I later realized that we fear a lot of things we would not normally fear if we kept our hearts and minds focused on Jesus Christ and not of our own desires. I was strong in my faith, so I was not going to give up, not yet, but I feared losing him. I knew I'll be alright, but he needed to be saved, really saved. Approximately two hours later, the ambulatory transport arrived with Rick who looked like death, a zombie, totally comatose. I have no idea what they gave him to quiet him down like that, but he was still, motionless, eyes closed, body stiff as a board. He was the total opposite from him screaming, cussing and hollering. He was alive, he was breathing, faintly and he was in a very deep sleep. Thank God, Sunshine was in her room when they brought him home. I was very emotional and afraid they sent him home to die. She walked into the bedroom praying, "You were born to love God, He created you. The Lord desires a relationship with all of us, but the condition of our hearts determines whether we'll experience it. The Lord can build an intimate relationship with you if your desire is to walk in His ways and do His will. Stay focused on the Lord and live according to his principles and in a manner, that pleases Him. Hold him close dear Lord," she continued, "be with him during the day and night, hold his hand, direct his steps, comfort his heart, relieve his pain, restore his health, renew his spirit, reveal to him that he is never alone, and that You will help him get through anything, today tomorrow and all the days to come. Thank you, dear Lord, for your favor, grace, and mercy. You know how weak we are. Thank you, In Jesus Name, Amen."

For He knows our frame; He remembers that we are dust. As for man, his days are like grass; as a flower of the field, so he flourishes. For the wind passes over it, and it is gone, and its place remembers it no more. Psalm 103:14-16

Sunshine, the prayer warrior stood over Rick reciting faith-lifts and prayers, "God made you so that you will glorify Him in everything that you do. Ask God to show you what needs to change in your life, give Him all your hurts and fears; ask God to guide you into fully trusting Him; ask Him to relieve all your suffering, give you the strength to get through it, and forgive your sins. We pray that God controls the minds and hands of all your doctors, that He will open your eyes, that He will lift you up, raise you up, align your organs, vessels, veins, limbs, wake you up, and heal you, in the name of Jesus, open your eyes, move your hands, arms, legs. Give him life, Lord, we know that all things work together for the good to them that love You, Lord and to them who are called according to Your purpose. Bring him out of his darkness Lord; allow your love to crowd out all his sins and troubles." Miraculously, Rick opened his eyes, moved his arms, legs, and was literally shaking all over like someone having convulsions. His leg flew up in the air and Sunshine screamed, "Did you see that?" "Yes," I said, stunned, smiling and in total amazement. Stuttering and shocked, I said, "Of course, I saw that."

And the prayer of faith will save the sick, and the Lord will raise him up. And if he has committed sins, he will be forgiven. Confess your trespasses to one another, and pray for one another, that you may be healed. The effective, fervent prayer of a righteous man avails much. James 5:15-16

He had not moved his leg like that in many years. It was confirmation that God was working behind the scenes. He opened his eyes and was trying to speak but nothing came out. "Lord, be merciful to us for we have waited for you," I said, "be our strong arm each day and our salvation in time of trouble. "God's people do not have to live in fear and salvation is a special gift from God." Sunshine interrupted,

"There are just all kinds of ways that God answers prayers, He operates in the most unusual ways with the most unusual people and He will use them in the most awesome ways. He can do it through suffering, bringing you to your knees (no pun intended), change your heart to know that you need Him. Wait on the Lord, He will not overlook your obedience so put all your faith in Him and leave all the consequences to Him. Pray with trust and assurance, God will work quietly behind the scenes." Rick was alive and smiling. He realized that his life had been spared and everything happens for a reason. Sunshine was a real faith builder for him. I had planted the seed and she was cultivating the crop. God is good! Thank God for Sunshine.

O LORD my God, I cried out to You, and You healed me. O LORD, You brought my soul up from the grave; You have kept me alive, that I should not go down to the pit. For His anger is but for a moment, His favor is for life; weeping may endure for a night, but joy comes in the morning. Psalm 30:2-3, 5

It was a miracle. God was performing His divine and miraculous interventions right before our eyes. One day at a time, I witnessed Rick build physical and emotional strength. I didn't think he'd ever be his old self again, but I still felt that God could turn this thing around. I would rather go through life believing God could turn this thing around rather than being on death watch. In the meantime, I would continue to help him with his salvation and keep him strong mentally and physically. Sister girl, Sunshine was a Godsend and right on time with her prayers, faith-lifts and a shoulder for me to lean on. We ate good and laughed a lot.

There are "friends" who destroy each other, but a real friend sticks closer than a brother. Proverbs 18:24

If I hadn't gotten it before, I got it now. I wasn't giving up but for the first time I was beginning to feel that caregiving might be bigger than me. I wasn't sure anymore that I was this superwoman that I always thought I was or that God had called me to be. Caregiving can sure make you doubt yourself and have you wondering whether you've done enough and the very best you could do. I looked to God to take care of me with his goodness so that I could give Rick the care of giving that he needed. I trust the Lord to guide me down the path of endurance. He held me up, held me down. God was the caregiver's caregiver. Praise Him!

Trust in the Lord with all your heart and lean not on your own understanding; in all your ways submit to him and he will make your paths straight. Proverbs 3:5-6

I meditated on God's promises, His word. God has made promise after promise and will sometimes go through the extreme when you really and truly want to know what his will is. It begins with the word of God, the word of God gives us spiritual life. This is where we find the will of God, in the word of God, so if you want to know the will of God get into the word of God. We have a choice whether we will walk in the will of God. He will show you what His will is. He has a desire for our life and He is committed to showing us what His will and plan is.

You will show me the path of life; in your presence is fullness of joy; at your right hand are pleasures forevermore. Psalm 16:11

157

I made it a point to spend more time with God throughout the day, often praying or just talking to Him. "I hope I can pass this test, Lord," I would say repeatedly throughout the day. Prayer is what kept me strong and kept me from totally falling apart, or bursting at the seams. I wanted to please God and be the best darn caregiver that I could be. However, sometimes, nothing worked for either of us because when he had a bad day, I had a worse day, but it still wasn't the end of the world, we still had our whole life ahead of us however long that was. We were living in times of uncertainty. Some days he did not want to hear music, and while his preference was to watch sports or old movies the television was often watching him, and it did not offer much to stimulate his mind or body like music did.

For He is not the God of the dead but of the living, for all live to Him. Luke 20:38

According to the Alzheimer's Association, Alzheimer's is responsible for approximately 60 to 80 percent of dementia cases. Alzheimer's often starts in the part of the brain that controls the memory therefore memory loss is one of the first symptoms of the disease. They usually start out mild and worsen over time as the disease progresses and spreads to other parts of the brain. There is no cure for Alzheimer's, but early diagnosis and treatment can slow the progression. Treatment for Alzheimer's and dementia is unique for each patient therefore seek the advice of a physician to know the best available options and always keep in mind with any disease or chronic illness, early diagnosis is key and because there are so many different types of dementia, it is very important to have it properly diagnosed and the first step to receiving treatment and discovering the cause. It is also possible to be diagnosed without a specific type of dementia, in which case the physician may refer you to a neurologist who will determine how to proceed with treatment.

Stand strong, stand firm, put Christ first, and make your life matter. Keep the faith, stand in the power of God, not man.

The causes may not be clear, however the effect it has on the brain is, and the brain literally shrinks. You can treat some types of dementia and if the cause isn't treatable, medication and other forms of therapy can improve symptoms and slow the progression of the disease so that patients can maintain a better quality of life and some independence.

And ye shall serve the LORD your God, and he shall bless thy bread, and thy water; and I will take sickness away from the midst of thee. Exodus 23:25

I continued to pray that love and time would heal Rick and his dysfunctional, nonchalant, and detached children that he loved so dearly, that they all would come to their senses and make amends. After all, they were only a phone call away. I prayed for love and a happy ending for Rick and his children, and I prayed that he could get them out of his head, so he could have some peace of mind.

Let not mercy and truth forsake you; bind them around your neck, write them on the tablet of your heart, and so find favor and high esteem in the sight of God and man. Proverbs 3:3-4

As Rick's end-stage renal disease worsened, so did his dementia and behavior. Although I'm sure the disability drivers in California had seen it all, Rick took the cake, and he took them through hell. Going to dialysis, he was fine but the return trip, he acted just like a pure-d fool, complaining, whining, screaming and yelling the entire trip home like an uncontrollable kid. One day he was fine and the next he was a screaming demon. It was irritating but he couldn't help it and he was unaware of his peculiar behavior. What could we do, we couldn't put a muzzle over his mouth. After dialysis treatment, the pressure intensified on his bladder making him feel as though he had to pee when he didn't. He constantly complained about having to pee and even though he had on disposable underwear he refused to use them. He wore them just in case of an emergency, but he never had an emergency or accident on himself. It was irritating and nerve-racking for the ride home, but once we got home it was all behind us. Thank God for working on me and my patience. I just may pass this caregiving test after all.

Know in all these things we are more than conquerors through him who loved us. For I am sure that neither death nor life, nor angels nor rulers, nor things present nor things to come, nor powers, nor height nor depth, nor anything else in all creation, will be able to separate us from the love of God in Christ Jesus our Lord. Romans 8:37-39

Today was a new day, and Sunshine was his baby sister. H asked her, "Why did Holly leave me here with you? Sunshine said, "She had to go to work, honey." He replied, "Oh, then what time she be back to get me? And, I'm not your damn honey. Why would she leave me with you, of all people?" "Because she didn't have anyone else to leave you with," Sunshine, replied, "surely, you don't mind spending the day with your little sis, do you?" He answered, "Don't get smart with me and don't you forget, I am the oldest." At the beginning, his mind would come and go and sometimes he would catch himself, feel ashamed, and shake his head in embarrassment. He was driving me crazy and keeping me in stitches at the same time, he went from one thing to another and from one extreme to another. There was never a dull moment. Rick was always such a creature of habit however slowly but surely, he became a totally different man.

For as we have many members in one body, but all the members do not have the same function. Romans 12:4

When I was a child, we called memory loss, "senile" or "senility" but that only happened to old people. However, while some memory loss is normal with age, dementia describes memory loss that is worse than expected at a given age, like in Rick's case who was 55 when his dementia started.

See what kind of love the Father has given to us, that we should be called children of God; and so we are. The reason why the world does not know us is that it did not know him. 1 John 3:1

Taking care of a dementia patient adds a whole other dimension to caregiving because it can be way more challenging and extremely overwhelming. He began to do a lot of screaming. I didn't know if he was in pain, constipated, hungry, all or none of the above. When he was unable to communicate effectively and unable to speak or express himself he would just scream. The sublingual Lorazepam helped a lot to calm him down and keep him calm, but it was happening way more often than I cared to give him the medication. Sometimes music calmed him and sometimes it didn't. His behavior was very sporadic and unpredictable. Some days he would scream all day and night and say hurtful things to his exes, referencing them by their respective names. It occurred more at night than during the day, but it could happen at any time of day or night. He was angry and cussing his wives out which was something he never did when he was in his right mind or at least while with me. The Rick I always knew was quiet, soft spoken, romantic, affectionate, kind, considerate, respectful, compassionate, loving and sweet. My heart really went out to him and I was walking around with a constant headache, no sleep and no energy. I just wanted to cradle him and rock him in my arms, but he didn't want me to touch him because he didn't recognize me as his wife anymore. When he saw me as his first or second wife, he would open a can of whoop ass and cuss me out like a sailor. It was hard to ignore but I had no choice, so I had to laugh to keep from crying.

But you, O Lord, are a God merciful and gracious, slow to anger and abounding in steadfast love and faithfulness. Psalm 86:15

Over time, Rick had difficulty doing anything. He loss everything: memory, vocabulary, appetite. He had mood swings, unhealthy eating habits (including playing with, throwing, holding food in his mouth and spitting food out). He was often irrational, sometimes disoriented; had trouble comprehending, speaking, balance difficulty (unable to hold things in his hand, or sit up straight in the wheelchair). But, the bottom line is he was still alive and no matter what I had to deal with it. I had come way too far to turn back now.

If there is no room for change, there is no room for growth.

Our lives had changed drastically over the years and I realized that our lives would never be the same. The dementia journey was real scary, crazy, cruel and brutal. It turned my sweetie pie, calm, caring and loving husband into a 10-headed monster. Dementia brought chaos, confusion and madness to our already complicated lives. Therefore, it made caregiving way more difficult than it already was. Rick eventually turned into a stranger, nothing like the man I knew and had grown to know and love so much. He really needed to be in a home where people were skilled and trained to treat people with dementia. Right away, you know within your heart of heart this is not your loved one, but accepting it and not being moved or emotionally affected by what comes out of their mouth and their behavior are a whole other issue, especially when this is a part of your daily routine. I honestly did not feel that there was any point of return. He had lost his grip and I was losing mine too. And, if he didn't know who he was, and he didn't know who I was, putting him in a home might not be such a bad idea after all. Enough is enough and yes, I was on the verge of losing faith, I was no longer in denial, I was tired, I was not giving up, but I was finally giving in to the idea that Rick was not going to be okay and I wanted to put him in a home because he was too sick for me to care for him any longer. He was getting worse and worse. I was losing sleep. I cried and prayed about it. I really felt as though I personally wanted to put him in a home, but the God in me, and my heart would let me, plus I had to do what I could live with, and I couldn't live with myself if I put him in a home. By the grace of God, the both of us would just have to endure it until the end and only God had any idea when that might be since there was no cure for dementia and it is not condition specific rather a group of diseases which causes irrational behavior and mental decline, affecting memory, intellect, thinking, and social skills which eventually inhibits normal activities. I totally understood dementia, and it was way too much for me. Rick got worse and worse so quickly and I was lost in the sauce as he became more and more lethargic.

I'm sure Rick was glad not to remember what he had been going through for the past seven years, he was able to finally block it all out, bless his heart, and I was happy for him to be able to do so. It was a very challenging time for me because I could feel Rick slipping away and I really wasn't sure how much more I could take. Thank God, he was now taking peritoneal dialysis, so we hardly ever left home anymore except for lab work once a month and I wasn't sure how much longer he would even be able to do that if he didn't receive ambulatory transport. He had disability transportation, but he needed medical transport. He would be sliding and darn near falling out of the wheelchair and I would keep having to lift and adjust him. Everyone came to us or no one came at all, mainly medical personnel came and went most often. Every day he was drifting further and further away not even wanting to get out of bed. I never thought he would ever forget me, but he had forgotten me a long time ago. I have never experienced anything like dementia. He could be looking directly in my face but seeing and talking to someone else from his past. That was amazing and a testament that his mind was playing some serious tricks on him. Eventually, all he wanted to do was eat, sleep and stare into space and if he was awake for any length of time, he would be talking out of his head, "pull my organs out, pull my pants off" when he had no pants on. I eventually realized that he was calling the cover pants. I had to be a mind reader too. He was often constipated due to constantly laying and taking pain medication. Nothing worked, Colace, Lactulose thick vanilla tasting syrup that he hated and would spit everywhere). I know this is gross, but I would put on a facemask and for however many days it took, I pulled huge hard poop balls out of his behind because he could not move his bowels on his own and would scream and cry in excruciating pain, so I had to give him a suppository and help him go to give him some relief. It was rough, and I went through a lot, more than anyone could ever imagine. He would not wear disposal underwear at home because they made him sweat and irritated him. They could also cause bedsores. He was urinating in the bed rather than using the urinal, so I had to constantly change and wash his clothes, mattress, bed pads and linen plus clean him up. I had OCD, so my house never stunk.

Oh, give thanks to the LORD, for He is good! For His mercy endures forever. Psalm 107:1

One good thing, his bedsore miraculously healed. I did exactly what they told me NOT to do. I stuffed the hole with gauze with aloe vera; kept him on a lamb's wool pad covered with corn starch, cleaned the sore with peroxide; and it eventually dried up and closed completely up. It was a miracle. The wound care staff couldn't believe it and neither could I. They said they had never seen anything like it. I was proud to have healed a stage four bedsore. They had always told me how clean the sore was and that it never smelled, and they wondered what I was doing to keep the odor down because most stage four bedsores had a horribly foul odor. I kept it clean because I was truly afraid of gangrene. I was also afraid that he might get an ulcer on his foot or other parts of his body next, so I used special creams and ointments to keep his skin moisturized. I was horrified of bedsores, but he was very immobile, so they were inevitable, like the doctor said especially if he continued to lie in one spot for too long. It was extremely hard for him to understand why his foot had to be elevated and why I had to turn him so often. He didn't comprehend much of anything anymore and it was rather frustrating because he acted as though I was being a nuisance and constantly disturbing him. He was basically filled with empty looks and blank stares. I had to constantly remind myself that he was not the Rick I knew or married, that Rick was long gone. Thank God for memories and memories are forever. I began to think about the good old days when he gave me butterflies, roses, wine and dined me, gave me beautiful and romantic Hallmark cards regularly, smothered me with love, hugs and kisses; massaged my feet; tickled my feet, underarms, and belly; and whispered sweet things in my ears. He was still handsome, but he used to be so much fun, dry humor but still funny and he was so kindhearted, caring and compassionate. Thoughts of the way we were always made me smile rather than cry. We used to be so happy. Those were the good old days. However, the bible says it is not wise to long for the good old days.

Don't long for "the good old days." This is not wise. Ecclesiastes 7:10

The next morning, I was happy, bubbly and jolly and as usual Rick woke up just the opposite, calling me his first ex-wife. He was very belligerent and short with her. I was too tired to be bothered today. I started massaging him, rubbing his legs, back and neck to relax him like I have done for years but I could tell that I was aggravating him. I just wanted him to be quiet. I tried kissing him and that aggravated the heck out of him even more. He was not having it. He said, "Witch, what are you doing? What the heck is wrong with you, do not do that, do not try to kiss me, don't touch me, you know I don't like you like that?" Backing away a few inches, I said, "Okay, okay, I'm sorry but I'm your wife, you just don't remember me. I'm sorry." He gave me a real crazy look. He set straight up in the bed, on his own, something he normally could not do alone, and he proceeded to spit in my face, while yelling, "You are not my damn wife, witch and stop saying that shit, you fake wannabe, you are not my wife, and I can't stand your dumb ass, so stop saying you're my wife, you used to be my wife, you are my kid's mother, that's all you are. You haven't been my wife for years and you never deserved to be my wife in the first place. Get it through your bug face, fathead, you are my baby mommy, two times, okay, that's it. I should never have married you, you treated me horrible. You turned my kids against me, especially our son. You kept my kids from me a lot of times. All of them act funny. You manipulated me and played too many mind games. You lied to my mother and grandmother about me and called the police on me. I accepted your daughter and she turned her back on me too." I was in a state of shock because I thought they were close friends but obviously not and the one I thought wasn't so close, obviously was. Now, I was confused. Lord, help me. I always played along with him because I did not want to do anything to antagonize him or make him angry or alter his behavior. After that, I just decided to stick to playing it safe and just go along with the program, no more reasoning or explaining on my part. I'm done. He called Sunshine everything from Brown to Ginger to his baby sister, I assume due to her gorgeous California bubbling brown sugar to bronze tan that reflected off her blond hair. I do not know how I survived without her, she would cook, clean and sit with Rick. God was really working in our lives, I was not feeling the stress nearly as much as I had at the beginning.

You did not choose me, but I chose you and appointed you that you should go and bear fruit and that your fruit should abide, so that whatever you ask the Father in my name, he may give it to you. John 15:16

Rick behaved very badly toward his ex-wives. There was a lot going on in that head of his. I wore a bunch of hats, including nurse, doctor, mother, grandmother, wives, etc. No matter what, I had to remain calm and not take anything personal. I had to practice what I preached because I knew "a fool is quick to anger but a wise person stays calm when insulted," so I exercised a lot of patience even when I was being wronged or mistreated.

A fool's wrath is known at once, but a prudent man covers shame. Proverbs 12:16

Rick hadn't changed, only his behavior had. He had forgotten me, but I would never forget him. He was still Rick, just in rare form. I did everything in my power to keep him happy, comfortable and not lose patience with him, but it wasn't easy. I had no choice but to be tolerant, extremely easy-going and open-minded but I'm not sure I could take another spit in the face. Regardless to who he thought I was he was my dear sweet gravely ill husband who had turned into an uncontrollable angry, crazed and combative maniac. But, my heart was genuine, and it really went out to him. As bad as his behavior was, I was still madly in love with him and hopeful. I did not know what to do but I wanted to help him so much that I started looking for a trial study for individuals with memory loss and dementia but there was nothing available for people like him except for a nursing home or memory care facility. I felt that even if he did not benefit from the study it may help others in the future, perhaps even save lives. God willing, I was determined to endure it to the end and continue to give him all the support he needed.

I have shown you in every way, by laboring like this, that you must support the weak. And remember the words of the Lord Jesus, that He said, "It is more blessed to give than to receive." Acts 20:35

Life was crazier than ever if that was possible. I was feeling burnt out again. I felt bad for him. All I wanted to do was help him like I have always done in the past, but I just couldn't anymore because his mind was going, almost gone, I couldn't reason or talk to him anymore. Some days he would scream for hours like I was trying to kill him.

Reaching Out

Caring for a disabled, chronically or terminally ill loved one whether it is a child, parent, partner, spouse, friend or family member can lead to a ball of confusion, and a flood of complicated emotions, including episodes of anger or bitterness, frustration because you expect things to change, for the better, with the quickness but instead things are up and down, and spinning around, all the time and for a very long time. Sometimes I did not feel like the wheels were turning in my life. I would feel guilty for becoming frustrated, irritated, overwhelmed, resentful and impatient. I began to be overcome by my emotions and full because it was just so painful to watch an extremely independent, happy, strong, resilient young man gradually succumb to his sickness and eventually be forced to give up all the things he enjoyed and loved doing so much. In my capacity as caregiver, I became emotionally, physically and mentally exhausted. I was totally sleep deprived. I do not know what I would have done without God.

Casting all your care upon Him, for He cares for you. 1 Peter 5:7

Sometimes I felt like I was drowning in Rick's sorrow because I did share his pain. I had also been a caregiver to my mother along with other family members and a few friends, so I thought I was strong and could handle anything. My mother was a five-year cervical cancer survivor, but she was a non-smoker that died from lung cancer. The following year, my niece passed away and I helped take care of her kids while my sister and her husband took care of her terminally ill daughter. My sister supported the children financially. Bless her heart. Rick became gravely ill the same year my niece passed away. Being a fulltime caregiver was extremely challenging and I came to realize very late in the game that I could only do but so much and that I needed help before I have a nervous breakdown. At least with my mom, it was several of us who shared the responsibility of caring for her. I think the hardest thing was asking for and admitting that I needed help. However, the sicker Rick became the more I had to do and the more helpless I felt plus that meant doing even less and less for myself. In addition to administering his insulin, Procrit or Epogen shots, I had to brush his teeth, bathe him; shave his face, ears and nose; clip his fingernails and toenails, as needed; wash and comb his hair, lift him on and off the toilet, wipe his butt, put him in the wheelchair, take him to the table, prepare his meals, sometimes feed him his meals, lift him in and out of bed, sit him up and lie him down in bed, pull him up in the bed and wheelchair – no matter what he needed, wanted to do or did, he was totally dependent upon me to do it for him, thus requiring my assistance nonstop. I keep praising the Lord for giving me that kind of strength when I needed it. It wasn't in me, it was the God in me. Thank you, Lord for being the caregiver's caregiver.

But the salvation of the righteous is from the Lord; He is their strength in time of trouble. Psalm 37:39

If nothing else, I had to at least get someone in to bathe him or a home health aide a few hours a week. That may not sound like much, but one hour a week would be a huge help. Anything would've be more than I had at the time. Thank God, my son and his wife were always there, especially since they lived only a few blocks away and eventually became our next-door neighbor. God, did it again! But, they worked and had a family. The Lord has been good to us, blessing us abundantly, despite all the challenges and setbacks we have had. We are grateful for all the comebacks.

171

Return to your rest, O my soul, for the LORD has dealt bountifully with you. Psalm 116:7

But, I still wasn't sure how much longer I could do this. I was so tempted to put him in a home. Half the time, I was out of breath, feeling, looking and walking like an old lady. I had aged 10 years. My legs were swollen and tired all the time. It was just hard taking the little dignity and peace he had left away from him. I did not want to turn his life into any more turmoil than it already was, so I had to do what I always came back to—keeping him at home. I knew if Rick went into a home, he would not last long. He was a spoiled brat, and it was my fault. I absolutely adored that man and I felt so sorry for what he was going through and the best thing that I could do for him was to keep him comfortable and make his life meaningful and enjoyable. We had cried and laughed a lot. I knew I was his everything and he was mine. I prayed that love could keep us together. If love can save him, we have nothing to worry about because we had plenty of love and love endures through every circumstance.

Love suffers long and is kind; love does not envy; love does not parade itself, is not puffed up; does not behave rudely, does not seek its own, is not provoked, thinks no evil; does not rejoice in iniquity, but rejoices in the truth; bears all things, believes all things, hopes all things, endures all things. 1 Corinthians 13:4-7

I remained hopeful and optimistic. When I decided to care for Rick at home I made that decision based on what I could live with. I could not live with leaving him in someone else's care 24-7 and since we had discussed nursing and rehabilitation homes before his condition worsened, I knew without a shadow of a doubt that he did not want to ever go into a home. He was afraid of being abused or mistreated, so it was his desire to stay at home and I had planned to honor his wishes to the end. Although at the time we talked, we had no idea how his health would worsen to the extent he had.

Pray that you may prosper in all things, health, wealth, mind, body and spirit.

Chapter 5

Faith Gives Strength

Some days Rick was upset and disappointed to wake up or face another day. He was just the opposite of most people who was happy to see the light of day. Most of the time music helped, other times nothing did any good. He loved playing games and me reading to him, but I didn't have a lot of time to read to him. When he was down in the dumps I was determined that he was not going to drag me down with him. "Better one man down than two" was my motto. Thank God, I had put Rick in God's hands a long time ago and glory be to God for strengthening and nourishing me spiritually.

Now Glory Be to God! By his mighty power at work within us, He is able to accomplish infinitely more than we would ever dare to ask or hope. Ephesians 3:20-21

Rick has been sick for many years and no matter how long it has been I remain optimistic, and very hopeful—I will never stop trying to keep him encouraged. "You open your eyes day after day, year after year, no matter what the problems or circumstances are," I said, "so you should live in vision instead of circumstance, choose to be happy, thankful, prayerful, faithful and hopeful in knowing that it could always be worse and somehow God will eventually work it all out. Every day is an opportunity for you to live, not be sad or on death watch."

This is the day the Lord has made, let us rejoice and be glad in it. Psalm 118:24

"My mom said, 'It takes over 40 muscles to frown and 17 to smile' so it just makes more sense to smile than frown," to make him smile, I said, "laughter adds joy to your life, it is good medicine for the soul and it costs you nothing, it'll make you feel better too. Trust me, God didn't bring you this far to leave you so stop looking so sad. Misery, happiness and joy are all choices. It's totally up to you. Stop making yourself miserable and sicker. Hold your head up high, not down because this too shall pass." He smiled and that's all that mattered.

Because thou shalt forget thy misery, and remember it as waters that pass away. Job 11:16

"Worry about nothing and pray about everything," I said. "I do pray but my prayers are not answered like yours, he said, "I guess that's why God gave me you because God always answers your prayers. You're a real earth angel." "Aww," I said, "you're so sweet, and thank you but God answers all prayers." I clarified, "yes, no, or wait—I pray, thank Him, trust Him, worship Him and praise Him all the time, I include Him in everything that I do, I live a joyful life and I have lots of faith; I also witness and try to be good to others. I treat people the way that I want to be treated, not the way people treat me. Even those who have wronged me, I do not only forgive them, I forget too. I do not hold grudges. The same things God does for me he will also do for you. I do not always get the answers I want but none of my prayers goes unanswered. Happiness and worrying cannot co-exist if you are walking by faith. Once you totally trust God, nothing else matters, no more worrying, that's for sure. I keep telling you that He will take care of you like a father cares for his child. I am Godspoiled and he will spoil you too." "Yes, you are Godspoiled," he cosigned, "and you are my angel baby."

And this same God who takes care of me will supply all your needs from his glorious riches, which have been given to us in Christ Jesus. Now Glory Be to God our Father forever and ever. Amen. Philippians 4:19

"Aww, thank you, that is so sweet," I said, "I am Godspoiled, but life can change in an instant, so I take nothing for granted. Everything happens for a reason and God put me in your life for a reason." I knew that God was using me to demonstrate faith, trust and humbleness. Impossible goals can be accomplished through faith.

Fix these words of mine in your hearts and minds; tie them as symbols on your hands and bind them on your foreheads. Deuteronomy 11:18

"You can be happy amid your storm though. You fight your fears and find your way back by walking on water faith, faith by grace will remove your worries and fears. Peter walked on water for about two seconds, before he allowed his fear of failure to be stronger than his faith in God, so he began sinking but God did not let him drown. Faith is a survival tool. I wake up every day knowing that it's going to be alright no matter what lies ahead, and I am not going to let anyone take that away from me," I preached, "God does some of His best work with the most broken people and you are NEVER too far gone or removed from God to be loved by Him and used by Him. God will help you with facing your fears and building your faith."

Give yourself entirely to those around you. Be generous with your blessings. A kind gesture can reach a wound that only compassion can heal. Steve Maroboili

For the umpteenth time I suggested that Rick join a support group for stroke survivors. Bottom line, I was all the support group he wanted or felt he needed so his immediate response was "heck no." I do not think Rick wanted me to speak, rather just be there for him, seen but not heard.

I say to people who care for people who are dying, if you really love that person and want to help them, be with them when their end comes close. Sit with them—you don't even have to talk. You don't have to do anything but really be there with them. Dr. Elisabeth Kubler-Ross

I was faithful, to God and my husband. I believed in practicing what I preached. If we only preached and not practiced what we preached, then it is nothing more than a bunch of flapping of the lips, a mouth exercise, going through the motions. How I lived and what I did every day defined and demonstrated my faith. A true Christian does not have to act a certain way, they reflect the Holy Spirit and demonstrates their DNA with Christ every day of their lives by their actions and behavior which is beyond reproach. We can make God proud by possessing a genuinely giving and forgiving heart, following God's commandments and witnessing to others. I was determined to show Rick how everything changes when you trust Jesus.

God knows your every need but he wants you to rely on him for those needs.

The Holy Spirit will give you all the ammunition you need to live by faith. Pray without ceasing, open and change your heart to know God's purpose for your life and you will come to experience new revelations and have a clearer spiritual understanding of who you are and whose you are. As you move into a more mindful alignment with God's purpose for your life a brighter light will shine all over you and throughout your mind, body, and soul, a light so bright that it will bring healing. Above those dark clouds, the sun is shining and at the end of the tunnel there is light. Keep walking on sunshine in your mind and you will see beautiful rainbows in the sky all the time. Meditate on God and his beautiful creations. Keep your mind focused on the living. God will bring you totally out of the darkness. Sometimes God does not take us out of the storm, He takes us through it. Some people experience it all, the storm, the flood, and the fire. No matter what, you must be victorious, especially if you are going through all three – keep the faith and never lose hope. If you are seeking peace during a time of trouble you must find a way out or learn to cope and seek calmness and peacefulness from within. You may be in the storm but don't let the storm get in you. You can count on God to get you through anything.

He calmed the storm to a whisper and stilled the waves. Psalm 107:29

Life in California was a blessing. Rick was finally living one day at a time.

Do not allow yourself to become bitter since harboring bitterness will destroy your joy. Your attitude is contagious, if you maintain a healthy outlook, you can raise your sick loved one's positive attitude considerably no matter what they're going through.

178

Rick could not get over the way he was being treated by his family. He cried, "Broken heartedness will be the death of me at the hands of my own children, they are so heartless, no emotions, no compassion, who would have ever thought it? My sisters and brothers aren't much better, either, except for Babysis, bless her heart, she's the only one that seems to really care about me and has made any effort to make amends after our mom passed. It is not my fault that she de-willed them." "Disinherited," I corrected him. "Whatever," he said, "it had nothing to do with me, it was my mom's money and possessions, and she had the right to distribute them however she saw fit and that's exactly what she did. I never asked her to leave me everything. I thank God and pray for you every day and ask God to bless you, my angel baby because I have no one without you. You do not have to do what you do, thank you for all you do from the heart. You treat me better than my own family. I honestly don't know where I would be without you. I could never repay you or thank you enough for all that you do for me and you've done plenty. I will never forget when I was real sick in Stafford, you took care of my infant granddaughter and me too, plus you often fed my daughter when she came to pick up her baby." He apologized for his children and family not helping, offering to help or calling to see if they could help. It only bothered me because it bothered him so much. "Life is not a guarantee, it is what it is, and people are who they are. We do not get to choose our family. All you really need is God. When we are down we have the right to get up since we have convictions and the confidence that God has placed in us that no matter what happens we can overcome it. People may give up on you, but God will never give up on you.   You cannot change others, only yourself so concentrate on Jesus, not anything or anyone else, pray every day about everything, and for everybody.   Prayer really works, and it gets you closer to God."

The wages of sin is death, but the free gift of God is eternal life through Christ Jesus our Lord. Romans 6:23

I reiterated, "We do not ask for our family, they are just the hand that we are dealt and unfortunately what we see is what we get because they are our family and we are stuck with them. We love them but we don't have to like them, we just all need to get along and respect one another." "I may not be the best dad but I'm sure not the worst," he cried, "what is wrong with my kids, yours are so close to you and their dad." "You do not have to try and convince me," I intervened, "you're a wonderful man and you deserve better. I raised my children to honor their father and mother. If I were their mother, I wouldn't stand for them to mistreat you, or any sick person for that matter." He was so sweet. I did not know what else to say and I thought it might be good for him to vent. It was always better for me to listen when he talked about his children. Children can be a very sensitive subject and I felt his tears could be healing so I kept quiet for as long as I could. In his children's defense, I did interject to say, "Some people do not know how to deal with sick people. Maybe they believe you're contagious; not as sick as you pretend to be; or as sick as you say you are. They may even believe if you've giving up, then why should they care? They could also be afraid of you dying. Who knows, what they believe or are thinking. You and your children have a horrible relationship, an unusual way of expressing love and a serious communication problem. I don't get it. You can't change them so you need to let God fight your battles for you. God will not only fight your battles for you, He will compensate you for all your struggles when you keep the faith and stay in peace. He will be there to get you through this too. With God, you can find peace no matter what the circumstances are. Allow your struggles to push you up, not tear you down. You are not working under the enemy, or to be defeated by your struggles or your sicknesses, you are working under God so do not block the angels with your lack of faith from doing their work for and in you. The Lord will not disappoint you once you seek His will. At times, you may feel temporarily defeated when something you hope for doesn't happen quick enough or you do not get the answer to your prayers that you were hoping for but just be patient and keep the faith. God will not desert you."

I have said these things to you, that in me you may have peace. In the world you will have tribulation. But take heart; I have overcome the world. John 16:3

Wait on the Lord. When one door closes, another door opens with something better. Trust and believe in God's promises.

But He will not go back on the biblical promise to give His children the best. For since the world began, no ear has heard and no eye has seen a God like you who works for those who wait for him. Isaiah 64:4

The bible guarantees joy and comfort. God has been there when no one else has. I know firsthand that God will do for you what you cannot do for yourself, so you must have endless love and faith and be at peace knowing that God will deliver you. The Lord cannot be overpowered. He cannot be outdone. We cannot do nearly as much good for ourselves as God can do for us.

God is able to do much more than we ask or think through His power working in us. Ephesians 3:20

He can do way more for us through his power than we can ever do for ourselves. He gives us the power and authority to do anything. He can make a way out of no way. God will fulfill all His promises. To receive God's promises, you must humble yourself. Think of you less; but not think less of you. No arrogance, selfishness, egotism, or narcissism. You must possess a good heart and think of others.

Therefore if there is any consolation in Christ, if any comfort of love, if any fellowship of the Spirit, if any affection and mercy, fulfill my joy by being like-minded, having the same love, being of one accord, of one mind. Let nothing be done through selfish ambition or conceit, but in lowliness of mind let each esteem others better than himself. Let each of you look out not only for his own interests, but also for the interests of others. Philippians 2:1-4

Never feel that God doesn't keep His promises and blessings, He wants nothing but the best for you. He wants to put you in the Book of Life, help you through your hard times, depression, disappointments, hurt, darkness, brokenness, broken heartedness, sicknesses, rejections, finances, bad luck and all your problems, setbacks, sorrows, troubles and your sanctification too. Help from God requires trust and faith, the will to live, hope and cope. God will give you the strength, endurance, godliness, character, integrity and opportunity to receive his mercy, grace, miracle, deliverance, sanctification, salvation, eternal life, so stay strong and in good spirits knowing that God gives you the authority to power forward no matter what because nothing is too much or too big for God.

A cheerful heart is good medicine, but a broken spirit saps a person's strength. Proverbs 17:22

The day Rick had the stroke was the worst day of our lives and the second worst day was when he had to start dialysis. That was the day his life really stood still. I remember it like it was yesterday. I told him, "God will put you in situations, and circumstances, but give you the opportunity to get the help you need. It's up to you to seek the help and God's promise is that He will help you get through it. Ask for God's help and seek His guidance. You need a cleansing that will help you become the person you want to be as well as the person God wants you to be. God predestined that He will make these changes in our lives. If you do not obey God, you do not trust Him. You will never regret offering your life to God, but you can really miss out if you don't and if you do not trust Him there is no way for Him to heal, sanctify or cleanse you. You have to believe that God can do what He says He can do. Touch and agree?" "Touch and agree," Rick concurred.

Have mercy on me, Lord, for I am faint; heal me, Lord, for my bones are in agony. Psalm 6:2

Sometimes Rick said the nicest things to me, he called me an earth angel and angel baby. He also said that I should be an evangelist, but that wasn't me, the evangelist side of me was the God in me, it was in my heart, God speaking through me, and His message was "love everything and everybody, action speaks louder than words, so show by your actions and speak the truth about how you feel towards those dear to you, even those who have wronged you. Yes, even when doing so requires personal sacrifices. Keep your conscience clear and live by God's principles. You will be blessed when you worship God. Jesus' blood allows you access to Him and not only that we are redeemed by Jesus' blood. Devote yourself to God the same way you have devoted yourself to others. Show love toward your fellow man by being genuine and kindhearted." It could not have been anyone but God. Sometimes all we can do is pray for a person. Our prayers move God but for Him to listen to our prayers we must sincerely strive to meet His requirements and live by his laws. I cannot think of a better thing that I can do for a loved one or friend than to pray for them and with them. Love, faith and humbleness are godly ways and God's way of life.

Humble yourselves before the Lord, and he will lift you up.
James 4:10

Salvation

We never know when someone gets right with the Lord, a person can get right with God on their deathbed, so it is not up to us to judge others.

Everyone may not be good, but there's always something good in everyone. Never judge anyone shortly because every saint has a past and every sinner has a future. Oscar Wilde

Normally I felt as though Rick had a radar detector, GPS or some type of tracking device attached to my behind because every single time my butt would hit the edge of the chair, I was about to sit anywhere, or go to bed, he would call my name and I would immediately jump right back up like a spring. I could never sit down or eat in peace. I would have to do things while he slept which wasn't long enough to get anything done. I decided to track down an old friend, Sunshine from DC via Buffalo who, coincidentally wanted to relocate and I was in desperate need of a friend, so she sold her entire apartment and moved to Cali with two suitcases, just like that. She was my nutty buddy and she was good company to have around to break the monotony of this very long goodbye, the same routine, day in and day out with no true break in sight for me. Everything was taking its toll on Rick's organs and body. He had gotten progressively worse to the point of no return, but I remained prayerful and hopeful. I sure needed a good friend.

Many will say they are loyal friends, but who can find one who is truly reliable? Proverbs 20:6

Sunshine took him to church, bless her heart, her loving and giving spirit—to take such a sick person plus wheelchair bound man to church. Priceless! That was not an easy task, but I would take advantage of that alone time and I appreciated every second of it. She did not have to do that, and I do not know too many people who would have. I have an attitude of gratitude.

Thankful people have no problem working for the Lord.

I was burnt out and Sunshine had become my saving grace, and I felt blessed to have her around. It was also nice to have someone around who knew exactly what I was going through. We prayed over him, prayed with him, prayed together and read scriptures to him. She told him how God sent Jesus in the form of a human to live among them; how He lived a sinless life and taught people how to live by God's principles; how He paid our sins in full when He sacrificed his life and died on the cross; how the power of death could not stop Jesus, so He rose from the dead. She further explained, "when we believe in Jesus, He promises forgiveness for our sins and eternal life and when you accept God as your Lord and Savior, God can remake your life, so you will live in God's ways and a life God is pleased with. You no longer have to be a slave to sin and death; you can have eternal life." She was good for him because they both were raised Catholics as children and changed religions. She was no help physically because she had a bad back but spiritually, she was just what the doctor ordered, just the medicine we needed, and she was very uplifting and a breath of fresh air. She was Godsend to help Rick with knowing that salvation is the most powerful miracle to His existence.

Salvation is eternal life. In a prayer, Jesus described the way to eternal life: 'And this is the way to have eternal life—

186

to know you, the only true God, and Jesus Christ, the one you sent to earth.' John 17:3

"Salvation is for everyone," I reiterated to Rick. He was going to die and there was nothing that we could do about it. I just didn't want it to be a bad thing. If he was, in fact, about to get his wings, I wanted his transition to be glorious. Also, I wanted Rick to realize that no matter how terrible his life seemed or how bad it may have been God could help him live and die in comfort. If nothing else, he could help him to cope with his current situation and moving forward he would have more peace in his life. Sometimes he felt so bad that he did not want to hear anything that I had to say. His defense was "you're not the sick one, I am." Sunshine and I just kept giving him a whole lot of doses of Jesus.

Please cleanse us from all sins in the blood of Jesus. 1 Corinthians 5:14

"If you know the Lord and have accepted Jesus Christ as your Lord and Savior you have been guaranteed God's love for all eternity in Heaven," Sunshine said.

My soul finds rest in God alone; my salvation comes from Him. He alone is my rock and my salvation; He is my fortress, I will never be shaken. Yes, my soul, find rest in God alone; my hope comes from Him. Psalm 62:1-2, 5

Praise the Lord, for the moment, he's listening and praying right along with us. Sunshine taking him to church was inspiring. All the Deacons and the congregation prayed with, for and over him. That was a blessing.

If you openly declare that Jesus is Lord and believe in your heart that God raised him from the dead, you will be saved. Romans 10:9

Hospice

It is a real misconception that hospice merely hastens death. Hospice care can take place in a long-term facility or at home and in some cases the patient can continue to receive medical care. Medicare and most private health insurers pay for hospice in full. A patient can start hospice and they can also terminate their hospice care, at any time. The thing to keep in mind is that Medicare and most insurance companies will not pay for more than one doctor, team of doctors or facility to treat the same illness. In other words, you cannot be on hospice and be seeing an oncologist or primary care physician unless you are going to pay for it out of pocket. If you have cancer and decide to stop radiation or chemotherapy, there is nothing else the doctors can do for you except recommend hospice to help with palliative care for pain management and comfort. Same thing with dialysis which is a form of life support. Therefore, if a person stops dialysis, they will more than likely die within three months or less and therefore need hospice since there is no more the doctor can do for them.

Hospice offers a lot: expert consultations, 24-hours on-call team, a physician and nurse; a social worker, counselor, chaplain, home health aides and volunteers. Other services may include respite care, psychologist, psychiatrists, art or pet therapists, nutritionists; physical, occupational, speech or massage therapists. You and your assigned agent remain in charge of medical decisions and you may continue to see your regular physician. You just cannot be on life support. When is it time to involve hospice? That decision will probably depend on the medical team and caregiver as the need evolves since a disabled, chronically or terminally ill person may not be able to make such a decision. If a loved one wants to die at home, in a hospital or nursing facility, you should call hospice to discuss your needs or to give you some guidance. Primary care physicians will also be able to make suggestions or recommendations regarding home healthcare, caregiving or hospice care options.

Although Rick never had the true hospice experience I did and if Rick hadn't been on dialysis, hospice would have been a good option sooner. I benefited by having a sitter for 24 hours which showed that they genuinely cared about me. I was surprised to learn that hospice was not only there for the terminally ill, but that they were there for the family and especially, the caregiver. I was ecstatic to know that they were there for me and I felt privileged, a way I hadn't felt in a long time. It was great to inhale and exhale. I really appreciated hospice caring so much about me and insisting that I take advantage of their services. So, when you realize you need help, hospice is an option. They are there to guide you as well as help you to determine what type of care your loved one needs, and they will give the caregiver a break too. I regret not calling them sooner because hospice can enhance, and sometimes salvage the last stage of life or halt the painful process of dying, and not necessarily rush death like I originally thought. Hospice also provides grieving support after a loved one passes. Overall, hospice is an excellent source of information so do not hesitate to contact them, they are earth angels and will help you in any way that they can.

Thanks be to God for his inexpressible gift! 2 Corinthians 9:15

It's Time

I could no longer run any errands. I could not leave him with anyone, anymore—not even for a couple of hours, not even for a short trip to the grocery store or anywhere. Those days were over. I could hardly shower, and showers were very important to me because that is where I did all my crying and praying. I couldn't even take a walk around the block. We could have gone together, but he refused to get out of the bed and he never wanted to operate his motorized wheelchair, so I had to do that for him too. I had the arms switched to accommodate his good hand since he had nerve damage in the other one due to the stroke, but he still wouldn't operate it. Again, Rick was just spoiled rotten and when I did leave him with someone he would have anxiety so bad that he would throw up everywhere and pitch a hissy fit. He was totally out of control, so I was confined to the house 24-7. It just wasn't worth going out to return home to such a mess. He was fighting, spitting, cussing, hanging his legs over the bed, trying to climb out the bed and screaming to the top of his lungs. I had a difficult enough time with him myself, so I wouldn't dare subject anyone else to his bad behavior, but he did not try half of the tricks with me that he tried on my grandchildren. I had his spitting and fighting under control if I was around. He was a bad boy and I had mastered techniques to handle him and his bad behavior before it got to the point of no return. After all, I created that monster and thank God, he had the utmost respect for me. Rick was my spoiled baby whether he remembered me or not. It was something about my voice—if I didn't raise it, he was good and if I did, he would put more base in his. I was boisterous

191

so I had to learn to be more soft-spoken. I just couldn't take anything personal and I had to watch my tone.

There is one who speaks like the piercings of a sword, But the tongue of the wise promotes health. Proverbs 12:18

All I could say was "God, please bless this mess." Just when I thought I had a handle on the situation, he began pulling, tugging and messing with the dialysis catheter, sometimes yanking and pulling on it so hard, practically ripping it out of his stomach. Just like a child, if I told him to stop, he would stop for a while and go right back to doing the same thing all over again. The hospital basically gave up on him and told me to call hospice. They made it sound so final. I had refused hospice twice before and by the grace of God we had managed to keep him out of the hospital but there was nothing they could or would do anymore, so I basically had no choice, and if he ripped that catheter out of his stomach there was nothing I or anyone else could do for him. The primary care doctor wasn't even communicating with me anymore, I assumed because I hadn't followed his other two hospice orders. "Screw him," I thought to myself, but I finally decided to have hospice come and hospice was quick to advise me that they offer long-term care but no life support. I did not want to play God and again, I had to be able to live with whatever decision I made. Rick was incapable of making any decisions for himself and if it were up to him he would have been dead a long time ago. I had a feeling that it wasn't going to be much longer, that it was time. We both were dead tired. He said he was ready but with the dementia and everything else that he had going on, I couldn't trust anything he said because half the time he didn't know what he was doing or saying. I was never going to be ready, but I was so tired I didn't think I could go another day. Since the hospital and doctors had totally given up on him I was forced to call hospice this time because I needed help with everything from managing pain to dementia, so the supervisor came right away and did her evaluation. The interview process went well and a few hours afterwards I was pleasantly surprised when a "sitter" arrived. She was there to relieve me, around the clock, so that I could go out or do anything my heart desired. I was being offered a break, but of course, I did not want to leave Rick, I was afraid he may have one of his anxiety attacks. Him dying, even crossed my mind but the sitter assured me that they would be just fine. She had more confidence than me and I could not believe it, so I took her up on her offer. For the first time in years, I went out with not a care in the world. I came to the realization that the sitter was better trained than me. I prayed, "Lord, have mercy and please, do not let anything happen to Rick while we're absent one from another. Thank you, Lord. In the name of Jesus, Amen." I left him in God's hands. I needed that sitter so bad, she was an earth angel, and sent to take care of the caregiver. I knew right away that the caregiver's caregiver had sent her. Praise God and bless her heart, she was God sent and in Godspeed. Thank you, Lord. Praise the Lord! I couldn't stop thanking and praising the Lord. Just when I thought I couldn't make it another day, I was rescued. I went out to eat. I didn't know what else to do. It was truly nice to go out, have a nice dinner and a couple glasses of wine and return to a nice, clean and quiet house. I rested without any interruptions. Rick was fast asleep. That was unheard of in my life. I took total advantage of that Friday night and I was excited and looking forward to hospice starting on Monday morning to help me care for Rick and at least to keep him comfortable and safe from hurting himself or anyone else. I couldn't wait because I was tired, frustrated, overwhelmed and burnt out, but I wasn't giving up, it wasn't over until it was over. Saturday, Rick and I had a good long talk. It was like he didn't have dementia. He was so calm and nice after sleeping for 11 hours. We were both well rested thanks to

193

the sitter. We talked about love, living and dying. We talked about transitioning to eternal life, his desires, salvation, and his destination being heaven. I already knew his wishes and desires because we had discussed them many times before, but it was nice to have him back, but he was still in and out of fully remembering and understanding, but we were able to hold a decent conversation, it just took him longer than usual to get his thoughts together. He was speaking well and comprehending too. He even told me "you're so nice, thank you, angel baby, for everything; you are such a sweet nurse, the best nurse I ever had. I love you, nurse, what's your name?" I couldn't help but laugh because at least he appreciated me and that made me very happy, but I was afraid if I told him my name it might spark a mood change. "Renee," my name is Renee," I said. "Wow, he replied, with a spark in his eye, "that was my wife's name, my sweetie pie, she was an earth angel and an angel baby like you, she was a good nurse too but taking care of me for so many years took its toll on her own health, I told her to leave and go take care of herself. I sure didn't want to be responsible for the death of her after all she did for me. I sure do miss her. She gave me inspiration and read the bible to me and she was the best cook in the whole wide world." Rick had become the best storyteller ever. I shook my head and we prayed and went to sleep. The medication had Rick behaving like an angel. He knew he was going to die, he told me to give his property in Virginia to Babysis, his baby sister, if I didn't want it and I didn't. "Just make sure my kids don't get it, they don't know how to appreciate anything or anybody plus they never showed me any love, they definitely do not deserve it. I'm going to show them my ass to kiss like they showed me theirs," he said. I interrupted him, "Please," I said, "stop thinking like that, let go, let God, don't start that bull crap again, treat people the way you want to be treated, not the way they treat you. Put it in writing." Rick's mother left everything to him and it did irreparable damage and darn near destroyed he and his siblings' relationships forever, so I did not want him to do his children that way. I explained to him that was an evil thought, that God is aware of our thoughts and he should leave any punishing to God.

So get rid of all evil behavior. Be done with all deceit, hypocrisy, jealousy, and all unkind speech. Like newborn babies, you must crave pure spiritual milk so that you will grow into a full experience of salvation. Cry out for this nourishment, now that you have had a taste of the Lord's kindness. 1 Peter 2:1-3

He said, "I can't help it." "They dogged me," he cried, "I will never forget how they treated me when I really needed them, rather than show me love, they chose to show me their ass to kiss, I cannot get over that, I just can't?" I answered, "You don't have to, this is a perfect battle that you give to God and in the meantime, you keep treating people, the way you want to be treated, not the way they treat you." It had been a while since he mentioned his kids, but he sure hadn't forgotten how badly they treated him.

Do to others as you would like them to do to you. Luke 6:31

So many times, I had convinced Rick that he didn't want to die, that it wasn't his time, it would be in God's time, blah, blah, blah. I began to think that maybe I was being unreasonable and selfish because I was the one who wasn't ready for him to go. I was just as afraid of losing him as he was afraid of dying. Finally, seven years later, and still not wanting to do dialysis, no quality of life, suffering with dementia and trying to rip the dialysis catheter out of his stomach, at last, I said to him, "it's okay to go, if you really must go, go and be at peace, my love. I know you're tired, restless and weary. The load is getting heavier and heavier with no relief in sight." I think he understood every word that I said to him that night. He hugged and kissed me, something he had not done in quite a long time. We both had smiles on our face and tears in our eyes. God gives power to the weak and strength to the weary.

He gives power to the weak, and to those who have no might He increases strength. Even the youths shall faint and be weary, and the young men shall utterly fall, but those who wait on the Lord shall renew their strength. Isaiah 40:29

"Come and get me, momma," he yelled, "I'm ready to go – he was calling his mom, grandma, grandad and brother, "I'm ready to go, come and get me. I want to go, let me go." He just kept repeating himself until he fell asleep. He was calling on all his deceased family members. I knew it wouldn't be long now. It gave me the chills and I broke down and I couldn't stop crying.

And God will wipe away every tear from their eyes; there shall be no more death, nor sorrow, nor crying. There shall be no more pain, for the former things have passed away. Revelation 21:4

I envisioned angels waiting to welcome him home. No more diabetes, no more dialysis, no more dementia, no more wheelchair, no more walking cane, no more walkers, no more medicine, no more tears, no more screaming, no more doctors, no more worries, no more pain, no more sickness, no more dependency, no more suffering, no longer bedridden, and no longer disabled, instead he is brand new.

196

People after death become complete again. The blind can see, the deaf can hear, cripples are no longer crippled after all their vital signs have ceased to exist. Dr. Elisabeth Kubler-Ross

On Monday morning, a few hours just before the hospice nurse was scheduled to start, Rick got his wings. He had a grin on his face. It was confirmation enough for me. He honestly did not want another nurse, hospice, or otherwise, he had finally had enough, and all he wanted was peace. He called where we lived in California, a paradise. God rest his soul, he really was resting in paradise now. Rick was gone way too soon, Lord have mercy, and Rick was gone. I wasn't mad. As a matter of fact, I was quite happy for him and relieved for myself, but it was weird talking about him in the past tense. Sunshine came into the bedroom, closed his eyes, and prayed. God bless his soul. It was time. I do not think I could have gone another day. God knows just how much a person can take and He won't put any more on you than you can bear.

No temptation has overtaken you except such as is common to man; but God is faithful, who will not allow you to be tempted beyond what you are able, but with the temptation will also make the way of escape, that you may be able to bear it. 1 Corinthians 10:13

I was obligated and committed to the Lord. Praise the Lord, I had weathered the storm, and by God's good grace, I ran the race, and endured it to the end. Glory be to God! I could not thank God enough for getting me through this experience, alive. Although it was extremely challenging and difficult I persevered. I came close to it, but I never gave up hope or lost faith. I hope I made Him proud. Glory, glory, hallelujah!

Not only that, but we rejoice in our sufferings, knowing that suffering produces endurance, and endurance produces character, and character produces hope. Romans 5:3-4

Before Rick passed away, I never really understood death being a celebration, but I do now. I endured it to the end. I'm at peace knowing he's at peace. He's in paradise, and I have an angel.

And he said to him, "Truly, I say to you, today you will be with me in Paradise. Luke 23:43

Chapter 6

Afterwards

Our lives really changed in a blink of an eye and no matter what, nothing could prepare us for death. After Rick passed, of course, I had plenty of time to reminisce and reflect on our lives. Caregiving wasn't all bad, it was hard and challenging as heck, a lot to do, a lot of ups and downs, a flood of emotions, confinement, total devotion, very time-consuming and not enough time in a day. There were great times before Rick got too sick and some good times even when he was sick, he was nerve racking but funny as heck. Rick was my habit and my hobby, so I had to find other things to do to replace all that spare time I had on my hands afterwards. I continued to miss him because he was the most constant person in my life for so long. I had to be filled with the Holy Spirit to give up my life and to become a fulltime caregiver. God filled me with Him and emptied me out of me. I could feel God's presence all around me, all the time, He was the caregiver's caregiver, for sure. God is so mighty, powerful and awesome. I still live in the home and sleep in the room where Rick died, and I have no fears, no ghost and no bad spirits in my home.

And this hope will not lead to disappointment. For we know how dearly God loves us, because he has given us the Holy Spirit to fill our hearts with his love. Romans 5:5

All Rick wanted was for me to be taken care of after he was gone and thank God, we took care of that long before his health totally declined. Everyone was asking me "What are you going to do now?" "I am a 'goal digger,' g-o-a-l, that is," I made it clear, "and I put my entire life on hold, so I plan to write, live and travel. I was hopeful that I could pick up where I left off. I am going to see what God has planned for me, and go wherever He leads me. I still have a lot of life left in me, God willing. I will write until my heart's content. Writing is my passion and it is also very therapeutic. I love writing because it takes my mind off everything else, so I will write myself through the rest of my life. What more could I ask for? I reiterate I live a life of staycation, a life of joy, health, wealth and prosperity. I learned a lot during this experience but most of all I learned that my purpose is to provide a service. Now, that I am 65, I plan to retire from the traveling caregiving role so that I can devote all my time to a community chest of books, distributing free books to children in my neighborhood, helping with adult literacy, and homelessness.

Love your neighbor as yourself. Mark 12:31

Rick being sick made my life count–caregiving, or should I say, "the   care of giving" which is a spirit of the heart motivated by God, made me count? Taking care of Rick gave me purpose, strength, testimony and more faith than I ever knew I had. It also taught me to take nothing for granted. Death ends a life, not a relationship. Rick will always be my husband and angel. I will laugh as we always laughed; enjoy the foods we used to love to cook and eat, smile, and call him by his old familiar name because it is still the same. The life we lived so lovingly together is unchanged except he is no longer here. He is out of sight, not out of mind so it's okay if I think of him often or from time to time, or not at all, with no regrets and no sorrows because all is well with my soul. He's gone from the physical, so I had to let him go and it was okay because absent in the body, means he's present with the Lord and it doesn't get any better than that.

We are confident, yes, well pleased rather to be absent from the body and to be present with the Lord. 2 Corinthians 5:8

Sometimes, I feel as though God is speaking directly to me. I felt special, a true sense of accomplishment and received confirmation when I opened the bible to:

There are many virtuous women and capable women in the world, but you surpass them all. Proverbs 31:29

"Aww," I cried, "thank you, God, but all Glory be to You. Thanks for the endurance challenge and Rick's wings. I could not have done this without you. You were the real caregiver and hero because you took care of me." My work was done. I was beyond overjoyed. The doctors praised me for my loyalty and for taking such good care of Rick. Rick praised me for being good to him many times during his sickness, but I did not deserve any praises because I didn't do it for Rick, I did it for God, the one who orchestrated my steps, gave me the power, authority and strength to do what I did because I often thought I was going to die before Rick. All the glory and praises go to God. Trust me I was just going through the motions, a vessel. God is the only one who gives life. I did not keep Rick alive like the doctors said, God kept him alive by giving me the tools necessary to care for Rick but God, and only God kept him alive and me too for that matter. As hard as it was, it was an honor to be entrusted with such a huge responsibility, another human being's life. It was a doozy of a challenge, responsibility and the experience of a lifetime that literally changed my life, my whole way of thinking, and brought me even closer to God and if I had to do it all over again, I would and without hesitation.

And so we know and rely on the love God has for us. God is love. Whoever lives in love lives in God, and God in them. 1 John 4:16

The only regrets I have are: 1) Rick did not want a transplant, and 2) he had begun peritoneal dialysis way sooner. Unfortunately, hemodialysis and the diabetes had already taken its toll on his organs and body by the time he started peritoneal dialysis. Considering how often I had to lift Rick's deadweight prior to receiving the lift, I am blessed not to have a bad back. God is awesome and can get you through anything and everything and keep you grounded. Rick used to call me "Zena the Warrior," but, I was blessed and saved by the caregiver's caregiver, none other than, Jesus Christ and our Father God!

But thanks be to God, which giveth us the victory through our Lord Jesus Christ. 1 Corinthians 15:57

Live with Him and walk with Him, have an attitude of gratitude, love and appreciation for God's tender mercies, love, opportunities, divine placements, and miraculous interventions. Stay strong and keep the faith.

Do not mistake meekness for weakness.

Ask yourself what you can do to restore humanity in the world. Once we become more mindful about God, loving, humbleness, sharing and caring for others, we will all have a better and more peaceful journey in life and if nothing else, we will learn patience, endurance, faith and love, on a grand scale.

Remember Nick?

Ironically, after Rick passed, my old freeloading flame from the past, Nick thought we could rekindle a spark that he still carried for me.   I admit, I contacted him on Facebook through his son, and when his son called me back, he said, "my dad went crazy when he heard your name, he said, hell yeah, give her my number, that's the love of my life, my wife."   I had given his son my number and before I could call Nick, he had called me.   He expected to pick up where we left off.   We did become phone buddies, and while he wanted more I had totally outgrown him, plus I lived 2500 miles away, and I did not believe in long distance relationships.   I did however loan him $275.00, and he only paid $100.00 back.   That was a turnoff, and in the end, I wrote it off, feeling sometimes you must pray and pay people away.   He was not a man of his word so after that I kept him at a distance.   From time to time he would call and leave me a message mostly saying, "I guess you in Cali, doing your thang, you never return my calls, your name is not Porter, your name is Ball (his last name) so take that crap off your phone."   When I returned home, back east, he came over to my daughter's apartment and I had to literally fight him off to keep him from raping me so that was the last turnoff.   He could have thought I wanted him.   My last communications with him on November 15th was when he sent me a text message saying: "You broke my heart and you wasn't thinking about me when you left me for your husband. Hooker!"   That was not the first time that he had told me that I broke his heart, but what shocked me was that he was holding a grudge for all these years, since 1997, this was 20 years later, and I regret not telling him, "I'll be standing on the other side of the bridge of forgiveness when you are ready." Rather, I said, "you were a crack and PCP head, and a jailbird. My husband, on the other hand was a very good man." Nick responded, "I may have been a jailbird, but your husband is a dead bird, so who, outlasted who?" I couldn't believe he said that, but he did. I responded, "You should watch your tongue. The devil takes care of his people too, and you just better hope you're not next. God knows your thoughts and everything you're doing."

My husband's anniversary of his death was November 14th. Nick's text me on November 15th. I was so hurt because I was good to Nick and I had vowed to never speak to him again after that disrespectful and nasty remark. We all must be careful what we say, and we do not have to say everything we are thinking. On November 19th, my niece called to tell me that Nick passed away the night before, Saturday, November 18th. I was not shocked, but I prayed that he got right with God. To this day, I have no idea how he died, an overdose of drugs, a car accident, a heart attack, another motorcycle accident, foul play, or natural causes, I just know that his name was in the Washington Post death notices and his funeral was December 5th. I also believe when you live by the sword, you die by the sword. I am still shaking my head because the statement he made about outlasting my husband was untrue. My husband died at 57 and Nick died at 56. I just happened to be a cougar when I was involved with Nick. When Rick and I got together, I never looked back and never gave Nick a second thought.

205

Grieving, Bereaving and Mourning

Caring for a disabled, chronically or terminally ill loved one can be extremely stressful and the actual loss of a loved one is often very devastating. After losing a loved one, we believe that we need closure and expect grievers to move on as if nothing ever happened. But, how do we move on after such a tremendous loss and especially when the person's life has changed forever, and they have no idea how to find their way back to the life they once knew, that they gave up, and lost so long ago. Where and how does one begin to explore a new life? We must understand the grieving and healing process first. Grief is an endless cycle, but it changes. It's a necessary process, but not a place to stay. While grieving is a natural and necessary process of loss, when you're ready to start moving on, starting new traditions may cushion the pain and allow you to take pleasure in attending or hosting special occasions and family gatherings again. Grieving involves many different emotions, actions, and expressions, all of which help the person come to terms with the loss of a loved one and since everyone's loss is different, everyone handles grief differently, and only you know what is best for you. Grief is the price we pay for loving our loved ones.

The five stages – denial, anger, bargaining, depression, and acceptance – are a part of the framework that makes up our learning to live with the one we lost. They are tools to help us frame and identify what we may be feeling. But they are

*not stops on some linear timeline in grief. Dr. Elisabeth
Kubler-Ross*

Just because someone says, "I'm okay" or "I'm alright"
doesn't necessarily mean that they are, especially if they
have not fully accepted their loved one's loss which is what
is needed to move on and complete the healing process.
Also, there is no right or wrong way to grieve and since there
is no roadmap to grieving it can be complicated and may be
very difficult. Although I was as good as I could possibly be
to Rick, I grieved just like anyone else. I had no regrets and
I didn't have a lot of tears to shed but I grieved hard.
Grieving the loss of my grandparents, father, niece, mother,
aunts, cousins and my husband made me realize that grief
never ends because you never stop missing and loving your
loved ones, you merely learn to live with it, accept it—and
the intensity of grief lessens with time. I have accepted,
healed and adjusted with the passing of Rick. I have
wonderful memories that I shared with Rick. So, while I
know that grief is a process, it is an extremely important part
of the healing process after you have lost a loved one, so
everyone should take the time to grieve because it cannot be
rushed, and it can get very complicated.

*The reality is that you will grieve forever. You will not 'get
over' the loss of a loved one; you will learn to live with it.
You will heal and you will rebuild yourself around the loss
you have suffered. You will be whole again but you will
never be the same. Nor should you be the same nor would
you want to be. Elisabeth Kubler-Ross*

When I reflect on the grieving process, I must reflect on the
experience of what got me to where I am today and how I
was finally able to accept my husband's death which was an
incredible loss to me and my family. The first step to healing

the grieving process is to honor your loved one's wishes and desires. You will have nothing to regret if you do, therefore it is important to discuss arrangements with your family—it is essential as the funeral affects them most directly. Usually the task of arranging for a funeral fall to a couple of family members or a single survivor who may have little or no warning. These people are most often unprepared for the many decisions that will need to be made. Pre-planning, prearrangement and pre-financing of funeral services should be considered before your loved one worsens. This will benefit those who experience sudden death as well as those who have more time with their loved one. Also, making one's wishes and desires known in advance can do a lot to help loved ones carry them out. Nothing can prepare you for death, but pre-planning will ease the burden when your loved one passes. Mourn, grieve, do whatever you need to do to come to grips with your loss. Blessed are those who mourn and grieve, and they are comforted.

To everything there is a season, a time for every purpose under heaven: a time to be born, and a time to die; a time to plant, and a time to pluck what is planted; a time to kill, and a time to heal; a time to break down, and a time to build up; a time to weep, and a time to laugh; a time to mourn, and a time to dance. Ecclesiastes 3:1-5

While grief can be complicated, you do not want to suffer too long since it is an indication that you are unable to work through it and move on to the next phase, the healing process. Complicated grief feels like a lifestyle and grieving behaviors are repeated over and over without relief. Grief without ever finding relief is not good and should be addressed with a health professional. Below is a list of complicated grief symptoms:

- Lack of energy, restlessness, and bored easily.

- Withdrawn from life, refusing to recommit, rebuild or reconstruct life.

- Unbearable feelings of guilt and absorbed with self-pity and self-criticism.

- Lack of sleep or disruptive sleep. Taking antidepressants, antianxiety and sleep aids strictly for coping with your loss.

- Frequently feeling exceptionally intense, confused and angry.

- Emotional wreck, sad and crying all the time.

- Being a know-it-all and in strong denial with a negative attitude.

- Unable to function practically and effectively with self-care, family, and occupational responsibilities.

- Lack of emotions, whether good or bad, pleasant or painful.

- Unusual sexual dysfunction or reckless or overly sexual behavior that wasn't a previous problem.

- Fear of intimacy. Refusal to commit to anyone or anything on an intimate level.

- Isolating yourself and avoiding neighbors, family and friends.

- Always feeling down and out with overwhelming sadness and a Debbie Downer all the time.

- You have an "I-don't-give-a-damn," "hateful," attitude, always being irrational or having an attitude toward everyone about everything.

- Lack of confidence.

- Constantly feeling discouraged and burnt out.

- Do not trust others.

- Need constant reassurance.

- Holding your feelings inside.

- Anxious, nervousness, trembling, or uncontrollable shaking.

- Withdrawn from life and feeling that life will never be right or the same again—and it probably never will be, but you should still be opened to rebuilding your life and finding happiness again. Happiness is a choice.

Allow others into your life or circle to help you accept the loss of your loved one. Family and friends are probably going through a difficult time accepting the loss as well.

Bereaving and mourning are also a part of the grieving process. Bereaving occurs when a person close to you dies and it is the emotional state of suffering a loss. Most employers allow bereavement time off with pay for the loss of close relatives. It is the outward expression of loss and grief. Mourning may also include black or dark clothes, ceremonies and other activities that are cultural, traditional, personal, and/or religious specific (candlelight vigils, prayer meetings, dinner, etc.). Hospice provides a remarkable bereavement program significant to the grieving and healing process. They host events to celebrate your loved one's life as well as offer tips on how to deal with grief and what to expect as you are going through the bereavement process. Rick was gone but hospice was still there for me, offering their support and expertise and I was deeply touched and grateful for all the services they provided my family and me.

After your loved one passes, it is a very crucial time to maintain the right mindset and heart. When you've come this far, there is no sense in giving up or having a breakdown now. It's all about peace of mind and what you can live with in the end, once your loved one is gone.

For God so loved the world, that he gave his only begotten Son, that whosoever believeth in him should not perish, but have everlasting life. John 3:16

I lost Rick, my buddy, my love, my husband, my BFF. Rick and I were together for a long time and he was sick for seven years of the time we were together. His sicknesses took hold of him like a whirlwind. He never really understood what was happening to him, so he must finally be at peace. I miss him dearly, but I was happy for the both of us on the day that he got his wings. We had talked about that day. As feisty and discouraged as he was, he still prayed to God to restore his health, renew his spirit, bring him joy, purify his heart, cleanse him of his sins, and deliver him from him health issues.

In my Father's house are many mansions: if it were not so, I would have told you. I go to prepare a place for you. John 14:2

He was a real sick man so all he could do was pray. Thank God, Rick wasn't mad, sad, angry, sick or crazy anymore. He was finally at peace and resting in paradise. He was healed, resting and waiting for the coming of the Lord Jesus Christ liked we had talked about so often when we talked about salvation and eternal life.

For the Lord himself shall descend from heaven with a shout, with the voice of the archangel, and with the trump of God: and the dead in Christ shall rise first. Then we which are alive [and] remain shall be caught up together with them in the clouds, to meet the Lord in the air: and so shall we ever be with the Lord. 1 Thessalonians 4:16-17

*   *   *   *   *   *

At Last

*Your sick days have finally come to an end,
My beloved husband, my angel, my dear friend.
Thank God everything has finally come to pass,
You have been delivered, you got your wings,
and get to rest in paradise, eternally, at last!*

Chapter 7

Pray with Love in Your Heart

We all could go through life anticipating bad things to happen, feeling sorry for ourselves, anxious, sad, mad, or worrying, or we can choose to pray and trust the Lord. We cannot have the Holy Spirit without God. Without the Holy Spirit you are helpless, hopeless, and copeless. The number of miracles that God performs is amazing and if you do not trust and believe, you will never know the power of God, prayer or miracles.

And a great multitude followed him, because they saw his miracles which he did on them that were diseased. John 6:2

God is my father and I talk to him like a child would speak to their father, always seeking his advice, approval and guidance. I let Him know how much I love Him and how much I rely on him and need Him in my life. The best way to deal with spiritual warfare is through worship. God knows everything about me, more than I know about myself. I asked Him to show me the way so that I can remedy or rectify any situation or circumstance. He provides all my needs and most of my wants too.

Therefore, my beloved brethren, be ye steadfast, unmovable, always abounding in the work of the Lord, forasmuch as ye know that your labor is not in vain in the Lord. 1 Corinthians 15:58

Besides, although I'm not His only child, I sure feel like it and I pray day and night, thanking Him for waking me up every time He does, even if I take nap. I pray a prayer of protection over my family, my kids, grandkids, friends, and myself even before my feet hit the floor every morning. I take nothing for granted and make God an anchor in all my decision-making. Every time I leave my home, I leave with the intent of doing a good deed or being a blessing to others, someone, anyone. When I fly, I pray for a safe flight and sober, well-rested, physically and mentally healthy, knowledgeable, and able mechanics, baggage handlers, captains, pilots, co-pilots, control operators, flight attendants and traveling mercies. Let everyone entering and leaving the airport be of sane mind and of no criminal intent, and do not have plans or thoughts to do harm to others. I pray that I do not encounter anyone who is crazy or contagious. I thank God for His protection. When I go to the grocery store or shopping in general, I ask God to lead me straight to the bargains because he knows what I'm working with. Amazingly, everything on my list or that I want is always on sale. Whenever, I leave my house, I pray I find it just like I left it when I return. I owe my life to God! He taught me how to forgive, forget and most of all, how to love, unconditionally. I love, appreciate and cherish family and friendships with all my heart. Everything I do comes from my heart. My love runs deep, I even cook with a lot of love.

For where your treasure is, there your heart will be also. Matthew 6:21

Do you have a godly heart? Do you believe in God's promises? Do you believe in God's miracles? How do you show love to others? Is it ever selfish, impatient, entitled, demanding or filled with the expectation of receiving something in return? God gave us the example of Jesus' perfect love so that we can model His love for others. What does the way you love others say about you? Love is what the world needs a lot more of and we all can start by being patient, loving, honest, caring, sharing, being kindly and witnessing to others.   Humble yourself, be kind, patient, loving, honest and preach the gospel. Most people don't know why they're here on earth and many eternal souls are in trouble. Share your testimony with others by telling them what Jesus has done for you.

However, Jesus did not permit him, but said to him, "Go home to your friends, and tell them what great things the Lord has done for you, and how He has had compassion on you." Mark 5:19

Patience and Endurance

Whatever you're going through and no matter what you're feeling, hoping or praying for—bible scriptures can give you a new and brighter outlook on life, give you a faith-lift, clarity, joy, harmony, add balance, and bring love into your life. Faith, strength, patience and endurance are essential to surviving the care of giving. This journey will be between you and God only, so feel free to use Him as your crutch. He may be all the support you have and need. Nothing can withhold the power of God. Dependence upon God is the best habit you can have so depend on Him, He wants you too and do not forget to thank God for his good grace for all He's done, doing, and going to do because God is the caregiver's caregiver.

And the grace of our Lord was exceedingly abundant, with faith and love which are in Christ Jesus. This is a faithful saying and worthy of all acceptance, that Christ Jesus came into the world to save sinners, of whom I am chief. However, for this reason I obtained mercy, that in me first Jesus Christ might show all longsuffering, as a pattern to those who are going to believe in Him for everlasting life. Now to the King eternal, immortal, invisible, to God who alone is wise, be honor and glory forever and ever. Amen. 1 Timothy 1:14-17

I craved more and more time alone with God—He was all I had. Sometimes I didn't want to talk about it or think about it and I didn't have to if I didn't want to because only God knew what I was going through and what lied ahead. Oftentimes I was just going through the motions so talking about it to others only made me feel worse or as though I was complaining. Talking about it was not going to change our circumstance so I opted to keep it to a minimum who I confided in and I did not like repeating myself anyway therefore most of the time I kept my feelings suppressed. Besides, most of our family and friends had already disappeared. I had gotten used to no one being around, so I wasn't up for a lot of opinions and advice anyway. Other times, I was too tired to be bothered. I used whatever energy I had to pray for strength. God answered my prayers every time. Enduring it to the end proves that God is more than willing to answer our prayers. Like I said before, none of our prayers goes unanswered – we just may not get the answer we want or was hoping for. Even in your weakest moments praise God because He loves and cares for you and will comfort and come through for you in Godspeed. It is imperative that we put our time in and take time for the Lord—be prayerful, thankful, worship and praise Him.

But thou, when thou prayest, enter into thy closet, and when thou hast shut thy door, pray to thy Father which is in secret; and thy Father which seeth in secret shall reward thee openly. Matthew 6:6

Have you ever felt as though you needed to pray, but didn't know what to say or how to say it? Have you ever cried until you felt weak, too weak to even pray, so you'd rather cry yourself to sleep? My mother taught me that when you are too weak to pray, the Holy Spirit takes over and prays for us so when you do not know what to say or how to say it, ask the Holy Spirit to help you pray just like you would ask Him for anything else or simply call on Jesus, call His Holy name, ask Him for help. You'd be surprised how They are working together behind the scenes on your behalf.

Likewise the Spirit helps us in our weakness. For we do not know what to pray for as we ought, but the Spirit himself intercedes for us with groanings too deep for words. Romans 8:26

Read a scripture, two, or even three a day aloud, when you wake up, when you get home, and before bedtime. You will not regret it. It will keep you uplifted and bring you closer to God.

For this reason I bow my knees to the Father of our Lord Jesus Christ, from whom the whole family in heaven and earth is named, that He would grant you, according to the riches of His glory, to be strengthened with might through His Spirit in the inner man, that Christ may dwell in your hearts through faith; that you, being rooted and grounded in love, may be able to comprehend with all the saints what is the width and length and depth and height—to know the love of Christ which passes knowledge; that you may be filled with all the fullness of God. Now to Him who is able to do exceedingly abundantly above all that we ask or think, according to the power that works in us, to Him be glory in the church by Christ Jesus to all generations, forever and ever. Amen. Ephesians 3:14-21

If you do not already know Them, you may want to memorize The Lord's Prayer and the 23rd Psalm. Both prayers will take you far in life and give you the strength, faith, power and authority you will need to cope with anything.

The Lord's Prayer – Matthew 6:7-13

And when you pray, do not use vain repetitions as the heathen *do*. For they think that they will be heard for their many words.

Therefore, do not be like them. For your Father knows the things you have need of before you ask Him. In this manner, therefore, pray:

Matthew 6:7-13 is slightly different than the one I was taught at 4 years old below:

Our Father who art in heaven,
Hallowed be Thy name.
By kingdom come.
Thy will be done
On earth as *it is* in heaven.
 Give us this day our daily bread.
And forgive us for our trespasses
As we forgive those who trespass against us
And lead us not into temptation,
But deliver us from evil.
For Thy is the kingdom and the power and the glory
forever and ever, Amen.

23rd Psalm

The Lord is my shepherd; I shall not want.

He maketh me to lie down in green pastures: he leadeth me beside the still waters.

He restoreth my soul: he leadeth me in the paths of righteousness for his name's sake.

Yea, though I walk through the valley of the shadow of death, I will fear no evil: for thou art with me; thy rod and thy staff they comfort me.

Thou preparest a table before me in the presence of my enemies: thou anointest my head with oil; my cup runneth over.

Surely goodness and mercy shall follow me all the days of my life: and I will dwell in the house of the Lord forever.

Pray without ceasing and develop an intimate relationship with God.   He desires to have a meaningful personal relationship with you that transcends all others in depth and richness. We must trust Him and relate to Him as a person. We often approach Christianity on a behavioral level by going to church, paying tithes, serving others, being a cheerful giver, being a good person, and trying to do all the right things God wants us to do. All those things may be beneficial but they're not enough. He desires more than knowledge and good behavior. God wants us to seek Him and know Him personally. God gives us free will. We have the freedom to make choices and God "wants all people to be saved."

I exhort therefore, that, first of all, supplications, prayers, intercessions, and giving of thanks, be made for all men; for kings, and for all that are in authority; that we may lead a quiet and peaceable life in all godliness and honesty. For this is good and acceptable in the sight of God our Savior;

who will have all men to be saved, and to come unto the knowledge of the truth. For there is one God, and one mediator between God and men, the man Christ Jesus; who gave himself a ransom for all, to be testified in due time. 1 Timothy 2:4

We have the choice between eternal salvation and eternal separation from God. Salvation is a gift from God, not something that you own. The devil takes care of his people too, but it is short lived – bottom line is with God you get eternal life and with the devil you get eternal fire. There is no other way to look at it.

Poem - Only God Can

Only God can
Have you confess
Bless your mess
Put you to the test
Turn a test into a testament
Guide you to do your best
Be everywhere all the time
Purify your mind
Change your heart
Keep you from falling a part
Change your heart
Sanctify your soul
Guide the steps of the young and old
Make a way out of no way
Turn a victim into a conqueror
Misery into victory
When life is upside down
Only God can
Turn it around
Right your wrongs
Keep you strong
Have you singing gospel songs
Only God can
Make something out of nothing
Make your spirit anew
Totally transform and transition you
Only God can
Really protect a woman or a man
Spread love in a country full of hate
Judge everyone entering the Pearlie Gates
Give you the hope to cope
Only God Can

Bible Scriptures

The Bible is the foundation for Christians' faith, the inspired and infallible Word of God. Everything we need to know in order to live under Jesus' direction is in the Bible. Will the decision you make honor God? If you are doing something that isn't consistent with the word of God or His direction for your life, stop. If it is inconsistent with the word of God, you are headed in the wrong direction.

One of the great things about love is that the Bible shows us a perfect example of how to do it every day and in every way. This perfect example is what John was referring to when he wrote, "We know what real love is because Jesus gave up his life for us." 1 John 3:16

The more scripture you read, the more dependent you will become on the word of God. You are never hopeless if you have God and He will work it out if you trust him. When you read the scriptures, it programs your mind to think, walk and act like God. His ultimate purpose is to conform us to the likeness of Christ. He is up to weaving and molding our lives, so our character becomes like Jesus because we are going to spend eternity with Him. He is your God and you need to be aware of His presence in your life. He uses us in proportion to how we need to be shaped. He is sifting out what does not need to be there so that we can walk in His purpose and the way that we respond is very important. Some people have been living in darkness for a long time, but they never gave up no matter what. When His will is fulfilled in our lives, a bright light will radiantly shine all over and through our lives.

Blessed is the man that endureth temptation: for when he is tried, he shall receive the crown of life, which the Lord hath promised to them that love him. James 1:12

Praise God for His mercies. I said "mercies," mercy after mercy, after mercy. My soul cries out for all the mercies of God. Living sacrifice is being alive and continuous in service, holy and acceptable to God.

So if you sinful people know how to give good gifts to your children, how much more will your heavenly Father give good gifts to those who ask him. Matthew 7:11

Lean on God along your caregiving path so that you will reach your destination in one piece. The scriptures are there for you. God never said that it would be easy, but He did promise to help you get through it. God develops us and makes us mature through trials. One or more of these bible verses just might get you through a difficult day or several days of trials and tribulations. Use them to your advantage.

This Good News tells us how God makes us right in his sight. This is accomplished from start to finish by faith. As the Scriptures say, "It is through faith that a righteous person has life." But God shows his anger from heaven against all sinful, wicked people who suppress the truth by their wickedness. They know the truth about God because he has made it obvious to them. For ever since the world was created, people have seen the earth and sky. Through everything God made, they can clearly see his invisible qualities—his eternal power and divine nature. So they have no excuse for not knowing God. Romans 1:17-20

It takes faith, trust, confidence, courage, obedience and commitment to live a godly life. If you are seeking joy and peace, look no further, simply read bible scriptures. Below are a few to get you started:

- 2 Peter 1:3-4 – According as to his divine power hath given unto us all things that pertain unto life and godliness, through the knowledge of him that hath called us to glory and virtue. Whereby are given unto us exceeding great and precious promises: that by these ye might be partakers of the divine nature, having escaped the corruption that is in the world through lust.

- Acts 2:21 – And it shall come to pass, that whosoever shall call on the name of the Lord shall be saved.

- Hebrews 13:8 – Jesus Christ the same yesterday, and today, and forever.

- James 1:2-4 – My brethren, count it all joy when ye fall into diver's temptations; knowing this, that the trying of your faith worketh patience. But let patience have her perfect work, that ye may be perfect and entire, wanting nothing.

- John 10:10 – The thief does not come except to steal, and to kill, and to destroy. I have come that they may have life, and that they may have it more abundantly.

- Luke 11:8 – I tell you, even though he will not get up and give him anything because he is his friend, yet because of his persistence he will get up and give him as much as he needs.

- Psalm 32:8-10 – I will instruct you and teach you in the way you should go; I will guide you with My eye. Do not be like the horse *or* like the mule, wh*ich* have no understanding, which must be harnessed with bit and bridle, else they will not come near you. Many sorrows *shall be* to the wicked; but he who trusts in the LORD, mercy shall surround him.

- Psalm 141:8 – But my eyes are upon You, O GOD the Lord; In You I take refuge; do not leave my soul destitute.

- Romans 3:10 – As it is written, there is no one righteous, no, not one.

- Romans 12:12 – Rejoice in hope, endure in affliction, persevere in prayer.

- Revelation 22:14 – If you love me, keep my commandments.

If you need additional scriptures, remember, all lines to Heaven are always open 24-7 so do not hesitate to include the emergency numbers below. Give God a call to cushion your fall and in no time at all you will be standing strong and tall, plus you will be forgiven for all your sins. Keep the faith and uncertainty will miraculously disappear. Trust in God and believe in His powers and miracles. The bible can come alive and fill you with love and hope.

9-1-1 Bible Verses

HELP WITH	CALL
Sorrow	John 14
Sin	Psalm 27
Danger	Psalm 91
When God seems far away	Psalm 139
Help with being bitter and critical	1 Corinthians 13
When you are lonely and fearful	Psalm 23
Paul's secret to happiness	Colossians 3:1-17
Understanding Christianity	2 Corinthians 5:15-19
Christian assurance	Romans 8:1-30
Dealing with fear	Psalm 34:7
Peace and rest	Matthew 11:25-30
Home Protection & Security	Psalm 121
When people seem unkind	John 15
Depression	Psalm 27
When the world seems bigger than God	Psalm 90
Help with selfish prayer	Psalm 67
Courage for a task	Joshua 1
Getting along with others	Romans 12
Empty pocketbook	Psalm 37
Assurance	Mark 8:35
Reassurance	Psalm 145:18

God Will Deliver

He will provide a way, in Godspeed
and provide all your needs.

Christianity/Bible Study	Emotional pain
Discouragement/Encouragement	Strengthen faith
Stress/Anxiety/Depression	Companionship
Low self-esteem	Rebellion/Lack of respect for others
Baptism	Chronically ill
Children-Parent Roles Reverse	Terminally ill
Temptation	Mental Illness
Patience	Alcohol Addiction
Endurance	Drug Addiction
Caregiving for a loved one	Stop smoking
Marriage counseling	Physical pain
Marital problems	Success
Physical/Sexual abuse	Failure
Death threats	Sick child
Forgiveness	Troubled Teen/Out of Control
Unemployment/Employment	Spiritual warfare
Raise/Promotion	Sadness
Alcoholism	Rebuilding life
Drug addiction	Rebuilding family
Spiritual protection/Satanic attacks	Anger/Bitterness
Citizenship	Death/Grief/Bereavement
Money	Diabetes, Heart problems, Hypertension
Insomnia	Stroke, Cancer, Heart Attack survivors
Christian couples/families	Unable to pay household utilities
Nightmares	Need food
Salvation/Sin/Repenting	Loan
Prosperity	Credit Repair/Paying off debts
New car	Pregnancy
New home	Wisdom
Homelessness	Legal problems
Home foreclosure	Fear
Traveling mercies	Death
Oppression/Bullying	Life
Academic/Business/Personal Success/ Achievements	Oppression/Bullying

Chapter 8

Caregiving

Caregiving is the care of giving that you provide to a loved one or the tender loving healthcare provided to anyone disabled, chronically or terminally ill. Caregiving usually starts out as a labor of love, but it can quickly turn into a huge and expensive challenge, commitment and a frustrating and overwhelming obligation. I advocate for family in-home caregiving. A caregiver must have patience and real tough skin because they will endure a lot of challenges. A caregiver cannot have a weak stomach, faint at heart, or be a weak-minded person. Caregiving is about giving up your life for another person, giving all your time and your life to care for another individual for what might feel like a lifetime. It isn't easy, not by a long shot, but it's doable, very doable, with the right mindset and heart. Caregiving is something that you must do from the heart; otherwise, it will be too much for you. It can literally kill you. Therefore, it is a necessity that you take care of you, as well as your loved one. Remember, the one the sickest doesn't always go the quickest.

Look not every man on his own things, but every man also on the things of others. Philippians 2:4

Also, do not leave the patient or your loved one hanging so you should never start anything that you can't finish. You must be all in or nothing. Everyone is not a caregiver and a sick person needs continuity and reassurance. If you have second thoughts, then it's probably not for you. This is not the time to doubt or question your abilities or capabilities of being a caregiver and while you may not be a caregiver you may be the only person your loved one has and when there is love nothing is too much trouble and there is nothing you wouldn't do for your loved one. Everyone may not have relatives nearby so in that case you may have to turn to others in your life, professional people, friends or neighbors. It is very important to establish a support network because it is extremely crucial to avoid feeling overwhelmed, burnt out, lost or discouraged. I encourage caregivers, family and friends to network and support one another. Stress and burnout can kill you and at the least, make you extremely ill, so it is important that you stay healthy so that you will be able to continue providing the kind of care your loved one needs. Find things that fulfill and balance your life otherwise you will find yourself sick and resentful of your loved one and if you are their main support system you will get tired, but you can't give up. You must come up with ways to make it work and to keep powering forward.

And let us not be weary in well doing: for in due season we shall reap, if we faint not. Galatians 6:9

When a person is stricken with a life-threatening illness or terminal disease, I know that it must change a person mentally and emotionally, but you never give up, you get up. I know everyone is different and I am not trying to diminish the role of caregiving in any way but caring for my mother was less difficult because unlike Rick my mother was not living to die. Although she was a five-year cervical cancer survivor, she had an aggressive form of lung cancer and while she knew her days were numbered she would do the best she could, and she relied on God, prayer and her support system to help her with everything else but she was not going to let man determine her fate, God was in charge. She never complained or felt sorry for herself and she was not a burden. She never let it get her down and she never spoke of giving up. She joked and spoke freely about death and looked forward to going to heaven. My mother wasn't afraid to die or talk about it. She knew the bible inside and out. She had an intimate relationship with Jehovah. She talked about her wishes and desires. At the time, I couldn't understand why God would have me or any of my siblings watch our mother die, but I soon realized that it was a blesson, a blessing and a lesson from God and His way of preparing me for taking care of Rick or anyone else who followed, although nothing could ever prepare me for my mother's passing. If nothing else, caregiving taught me a lot of patience, brought me closer to God and it gave us some extra special bonding time with my mother that we needed and enjoyed immensely. It was another one of God's miraculous interventions because at the beginning I told my mother I did not want to be on death watch with her and she told me that was too bad, and it wasn't about me, but about her and that was the end of that. I joined the team of caregivers and was glad that I did because the time I spent with her before she passed was invaluable.

For I reckon that the sufferings of this present time are not worthy to be compared with the glory which shall be revealed in us. Romans 8:18

I wasn't just my husband's caregiver, I was his voice, advocate, best friend, wife, chef, nurse, eyes, ears legs, arms, I was his life, his everything and I had to do everything for him. I realize that it's a heavy burden for anyone to bear when they receive a life-threatening prognosis but most of the weight still falls on the caregiver. A seriously ill or

terminally ill loved one does not only affect the sick person
but it affects everyone, the entire family and the worst and
most painful thing of all is that no one wants to be bothered
with a sick person, so he wasn't the only one suffering or
hurting. It was an extremely hard and lonely road for me
too, a road that neither of us understood, at first, one that we
were not ready for, and we had no idea where it would take
us. The first sign of the changing road ahead began when
we experienced isolation from our friends who began to fade
away from our lives slowly but surely, perhaps due to a lack
of understanding, we couldn't hang out like we used to; no
one wanted to travel the distance to where we lived; inability
to deal with the situation or sickness; and/or unable to face
the possibility of losing him. I have no idea what it was, but
it had us in our feelings, and had us feeling like we were
contagious or something. Family eventually became just as
scarce as friends. Rick and I often talked about moving to a
secluded island, since it was only he and I anyway most of
the time. Our social calendar was replaced by dialysis and
doctor's appointments and we stayed at home mostly
watching television, movies, listening to music, and trying
to adjust to our hospital-like environment, at home.

*For whatsoever things were written aforetime were written
for our learning, that we through patience and comfort of
the scriptures might have hope. Romans 15:4*

No one should take on such a responsibility as caregiving
unless they are serious and prepared to go the distance and
in most cases, the ride will be long and hard, and the only
thing that you can do as a caregiver is the best you can. You
don't know if you can do it until you do it, so be up for the
challenge because it will prove to be one of the most
purpose-driven, spiritually meaningful experiences, and
challenges in your life – it's huge – being responsible for

another human being's life, it takes a special person, and it's a "Jesus Calling".

I strongly urge caregivers to speak early on with their loved ones as well as their family, especially their children to educate them about the challenges and concerns such as home modification, possible role reversal, and long-term care before their symptoms worsen. Rather than wait until a crisis occurs, advance preparation, communication, research and visits to nursing homes to see what they offer and whether it would be the best fit could save the family and caregiver a lot of time and unnecessary stress in the long run, as well as help them to honor their loved one's wishes and desires which is so important in the end.

If you are a caregiver, do not hesitate to ask for help. It's a real test. I almost killed myself trying to do it alone. For some odd reason the caregiver feels guilty or like a failure if they ask for help. You are not and should not be expected to do it all, and while you think that you can, you cannot, you should not, and it isn't fair for you to do it alone. Make God your companion and comforter because He gives us spiritual gifts. The Holy Spirit itself speaks to us and will enable you to do anything. God knows exactly where you are in every moment of your life and He's there with you, to help you get through it all but ask for help when the need arise. Caregivers are usually some of God's toughest soldiers; it is an act of God. Caregiving will send you through a torrent of emotions and it will make a true believer out of you, have you calling on Jesus and you will grow to love the Lord. Again, caregiving is a "Jesus Calling" and God is the caregiver's caregiver.

Oftentimes, the caregiver feels like a nurse because of the huge undertaking and responsibility but with God being by your side as the caregiver's caregiver it will give you hope to cope, faith, tools, understanding, direction and love like you have never experienced before. Caregiving is a blesson of a lifetime. If a caregiving opportunity comes your way, don't dread it, embrace it!

Caregiver's Rights

- Being a caregiver is only a part of our life, and should not be your whole life so take a break, walk, exercise, meditate, meet and visit with friends, read a good book, take up a hobby, just do not forget about you and the things that you enjoy in life.

- You are just as important as the loved one that you are caring for so take care of yourself, first and foremost. Get a yearly physical and keep all doctor appointments.

- Feeling overwhelmed, frustrated and resentful is natural.

- Protect your individuality and your right for sustainability once your help is no longer needed.

- Seek, expect and demand help from family, friends, neighbors, and/or professionals to develop a strong support team.

- Find lifesaving outlets, pursue the things that renew you, create boundaries between love and independence, and incorporate a spiritual journey into your lifestyle and care. It is crucial for the caregiver to have a separate life, one outside of the person they are caring for.

- Maintain good time management to avoid becoming burnt out.

- Feel free to express your emotions and feelings, including anger and depression if that is what you are experiencing. Keep lines of communication open with family.

- Disallow any manipulation by others or negative outside influences.

- Avoid family drama; you have enough to contend with.

- Recognize the value of your contribution as a caregiver.

- Refuse to feel guilty or live with regret about anything when you know you are doing your best.

- Take pride in your accomplishments. Applaud your courage, patience, dedication, devotion and endurance.

- Find available resources, and support groups for caregivers.

- Laugh despite the circumstances and chaos in your life. Laughter is good medicine for the soul. It takes 17 muscles to smile and 40 to frown.

Helpful Tips

- The key to success for family caregivers is organization. Being organized will help you better manage all the different aspects of caregiving from medication regimens to having the right questions ready for doctor appointments.

- Keep a three-ring binder containing the patient's list of medications (dosages with number of times taken daily), lab reports, hospital stays, surgeries, procedures, treatments, medical records/reports, doctor appointments, Medicaid, Medicare, primary and secondary insurance information and payments, physicians, specialists, and family members contact information.

- Keep a typed list of medications with the dosage, purpose and time administered. Always keep this list with you. A list of meds should be on your patient or in the patient's emergency survival kit or purse along with meds and personal information as well as contact information of caregiver and next of kin in the event you two are separated during an earthquake, hurricane, tornado, flood, fire, etc.

- www.drugs.com/app is a free Drug.com health tracker medication guide app, available for caregivers and patients to download to keep a list of medications, reminders, obtain information, identify pills, check interactions, and set up personal medication records.

- Thousands of caregivers and patients also use MyMedSchedule to make it easier to communicate with their health care providers, track their health, manage and maintain their meds, vital signs and labs on the go, medication schedules, and reminders.

- Purchase necessary tools to record vital signs: a scale, blood pressure monitoring machine, odometer (oxygen level), statoscope (heart rates and rhythm), thermometer (take temperature to be sure there is no unforeseen infection); and if your loved one is a diabetic, of course, you need monitor, testing strips and stick pins.

- Listen to soothing music as well as the patient's favorite music for inspiration and brain stimulation, especially for the terminally ill (cancer, dementia and Alzheimer's patients).

- If the patient is oxygen dependent, check out the different options for lightweight, portable and concentrated oxygen machines with backups and capacity for storing oxygen in case of emergency, electric blackouts and traveling. Most of them are covered by Medicare once the patient meets their requirements with an oxygen level of 82 or less.

- If you feel the patient requires a wheelchair, talk to his/her primary care physician who may or may not agree because they may feel it is too soon for the patient to become wheelchair dependent or lose mobility altogether.

- Thermometer – TempaDot is a good disposable thermometer or you can always buy a digital thermometer but the TempaDot's are paper strips, and are easy to read and can be disposed of after each use. They are made by 3M and are sold in boxes of 100.

- If patient is nauseated have them sniff an alcohol pad.

- If the patient is having heart palpitation, have them do breathing and coughing exercises.

- If the patient has a problem swallowing pills, crush them and put them in apple sauce or yogurt.

- If the patient is constipated give them some flaxseed and a strong cup of green tea.

- To lower blood pressure naturally, take deep breaths in cycles of six. Inhale six and exhale four to six. Repeat this several times. Do not substitute breathing exercises for medication.

- Watching a fireplace burning and listening to its crackling sound can also lower the blood pressure about five points, as well as watching an aquarium, and classical or soothing music.

- Prepare a survival kit with a first aid kit, medications, dried foods, can foods, protein bars, water, soups and fruits, list of medications, emergency contact information, portable can opener and list of household members and phone numbers.

- If the patient is on a lot of meds, try to obtain a pill holder (preferably a 7-day, 4 times a day with morning, noon, evening and bedtime) so that you can prepare medication for the entire week. It will help you to remember what has or has not been administered daily as well as know what meds are running low and needs to be refilled. Also, the meds will always be ready especially in case of an emergency. Take advantage of your local pharmacy's prescription refill courtesy reminder calls and home delivery service.

- Keep at least a 90-day supply of medication on hand so you will be prepared in the event of an emergency.

- Purchase a few extra pillows for rotating and propping up bedridden or non-weight bearing patients to avoid bedsores, ulcers and achy bones. Elevate patient's feet by keeping them off the bed or by hanging them over a pillow to avoid sores and ulcers.

- Move patient from the bed to a chair for a few hours daily, if possible. Take them outside if they are able.

- Learn to properly lift and pull patient up in the bed. Ask a nurse or nurse's assistant to help you with pulling the patient up when they arrive and before they leave. Also, ask them to show you how to do it properly so that you can keep your loved one comfortable, and avoid causing injury to yourself or your loved one.

- If the patient is wheelchair bound, non-weight bearing or bedridden, speak with their primary care doctor about a lift. The lift is also good for changing the bed and moving the patient from the bed to the chair and wheelchair.

- If you do not have a lift, and you must move the patient from the bed to the wheelchair or vice versa, you can lift the patient by his/her pants (not the most comfortable way) or lift him/her securely under the arms and move him/her like you are dancing with them, just hold on tight and don't let go and do not trip.

- If the patient ever falls out of bed, or falls in general, call 911; do not attempt to lift the patient yourself. You could do more harm to the patient as well as yourself.

- If the patient is on oxygen, be sure to display an oxygen sign in the front window so that emergency personnel will be aware of the oxygen before entering the home.

- For easy dressing, particularly for bedridden patients, cut a 10-12 inch slit up the back of a T-shirt or any pullover shirts so that it can be pulled over the patient's head with ease as opposed to wrestling, tossing, tugging, pulling up and down, and making the patient uncomfortable and miserable throughout the day, trying to get a shirt over their head or from rising. It will remain in place, not rising or needing constant pulling up or down throughout the day and night.

- Dispose of any blood products in the proper receptacles.

- Stock up on disinfects. Always maintain a clean environment for the patient and others to avoid staph and other bacteria-borne infections as well as unpleasant odors.

- Use strong cleaning solutions sparingly taking into consideration a patient's sensitivity to the smell of chemicals, perfumes, fragrances, ammonia, and bleach.

- Report any change in the patient's health to the doctor or health professional immediately to avoid further health complications.

- If the patient is not bedridden, enroll them in a support group that they can identify with.

- Sign up for disability transportation with wheelchair accessibility, if necessary, and if the patient is bedridden seek home-health and ambulatory transportation.

- Locate an ADA transportation service if your loved one is disabled. Get the necessary placard and/or handicap parking permits.

- Be sure to keep life insurance current and keep all important papers in a safe, fireproof and easily accessible location.

- Talk about the patient's desires and wishes before their condition worsens and they are unable to.

- Prepare a Will, Advance Directive and Power of Attorney so that the caregiver can make medical and financial decisions when the patient becomes unable to.

- The patient may not be able to go out, but you can always bring family and friends to them. Have a potluck Saturday or Sunday breakfast, brunch, lunch, dinner or even dessert party.

- Designate a family member, friend or neighbor who lives nearby to check-in on the patient and caregiver periodically.

- Elderly people become targets and are vulnerable to all sorts of crimes so be sure that individuals do not move in on them, frighten them, take over their homes, abuse them, take advantage of them, neglect or steal from them.

- Set up a checking account which require two signatures every time a check is written and/or cashed if you or your loved one are unable to handle the household finances.

- If the patient is on life support, contact your local utilities company to make them aware. Most of them will give you a discount and check on the patient by phone if the electricity, water or gas is interrupted for any reason.

- Keep a list of emergency and family contacts on your refrigerator.

- Keep the patient's skin moist to avoid cuts, bruises, chafing and dry skin.

- Keep hand sanitizer with aloe and vitamin E and incontinent skin cleanser handy but use soap for sensitive skin and water as often as you can.

- Purchase dry wash shampoo or hair caps for patients who are bedridden to use in between normal washes because you do not want to wet their hair too often and cause them to catch a head cold, sinus infection, upper respiratory infection or pneumonia.

- Stock up on wipes, disposable wash cloths, body washes, oils, lotions, mouth wash, diapers, wipes, bed pads, alcohol, peroxide and lamb's wool bed pads especially for patients confined to the bed or wheelchair.

- Learn to make the bed with the patient in it. A nurse or CNA will be more than happy to teach you how to change the bed without moving the patient out of the bed.

- Do not isolate the patient from you and others. If they are asleep, it is okay for them to be alone but when they are awake, try to soothe them, be attentive and keep their company; have someone else sit with them; or bring them into the area where you or others are.

- Read to the patient just so that they can hear a familiar voice and feel the presence of someone in the room with them. Some patients may want you to just sit in the room with them and say absolutely nothing.

- Some patients want the TV on for company and others cannot stand the sound of the TV, so know your loved one's likes and dislikes.

- When leaving them explain that you'll be right back, that you must cook, clean, go to the bathroom, wash clothes, etc. You never want them to feel alone.

- For dementia and Alzheimer's patients, keep in mind that your loved may have forgotten you, but you have not forgotten them.

Are Caregivers Paid?

Almost all caregivers want to know, "Can I get paid as a caregiver?" "Maybe," is the answer since it depends on where you live. In most states, everyone can get paid as a caregiver except for a spouse. There are several options available, so it is imperative that you research the requirements and qualifications for your county and state programs.

Some counties and/or states have programs that help people pay for the caregiver of their choice, and in certain situations that can be a family member. These programs, varies in names and vastly differ depending on where you live. Most of the programs have income and other qualifying requirements that the patient must meet, and strict guidelines often apply as to who can be paid for the caregiving. For information about what's available in your state, contact your local Medicaid, geriatric or aging services department or go to the National Resource Center for Participant-Directed Services. There are usually long waiting lists for these types of programs and some states may have made budget cuts, so be sure to visit your state's website to see what programs are available.

Caregiver Contracts

If your loved one has some savings or other assets, they may be able to work out a caregiver contract to pay a family member or close family friend for their time and the care they provide. Consult an eldercare lawyer to make sure that any caregiver contracts you sign meets tax requirements, inheritances, if any, and is approved by all other interested parties (siblings, children, etc.). Be mindful of the emotional downsides of this arrangement (employing a family member or close friend as your loved one's caregiver can sometimes be too close for comfort).

Background Checks

You should always do a background check on individuals that will be working with you, your loved ones, and in your loved one's home – especially if you are uncomfortable or not used to strangers coming and going. Do whatever you need to do to ensure the safety and protection of you and your loved one. Avoid putting yourself in harm's way because at the beginning your home will be like a revolving door and normally you can trust everyone, but you never know so just be careful and keep it professional. Most agencies have already performed background checks on their employees but inquire to be certain and safe.

AARP Caregiving Resource Center

AARP has a Caregiving Resource Center at 877-333-5885 and website, www.aarp.org/caregiving.com that provides resources, tools, and support for family caregivers.

Home Care Coverage

If you have coverage for home care, you need to consider whether you have to use an agency or hire an independent caregiver. Obtain a list of facilities, so you can determine the places the policy covers and if the policy covers assisted living, be sure it covers both the care you receive and the housing costs.

Hardship Options

If you are facing a financial hardship because of a caregiving situation, here are some other options to consider:

- Eldercare Locator – www.benefitscheckup.com, check to see what senior benefits your loved one is eligible for and the eligibility requirements for programs that may provide an outside caregiver, so the responsibility doesn't fall solely on the caregiver.

- If you must work, consider finding work you can do at home, or find a job that allows you the flexibility you need to be a caregiver which is much easier said than done.

- Hold a family meeting with siblings and others to discuss ways you can all share the financial burden and caregiving responsibilities.

- Remember your financial, mental, physical and emotional well-being should remain a top priority so that you may continue to provide the kind of care your loved one needs.

- Inquire as to whether the Federal Leave Act could benefit the working caregiver or other family members that may be able to provide support.

Probably way more Americans than we can imagine provide care for an elderly, disabled, chronically or terminally ill loved one.   Some of the more fortunate caregivers can benefit from the Federal Leave Act, while it's a balancing act between work and home for many others.   And, even those with the Federal benefit, must have leave to fully benefit from it and most people with a sick parent or loved one has already exhausted all their leave with doctor appointments, treatments, hospital stays, etc.

Veterans' Benefits

A law passed in 2010 provides a monthly stipend to primary caregivers of veterans injured in military conflict after 9/11. Other benefits to caregivers include travel expenses, access to health care insurance, mental health services and respite care of 30 days a year.   For more information, call the Department of Veterans Affairs at 1-877-222-VETS (8387). Some state programs are specifically geared toward veterans. In addition, the VA also has available a VA's Aid and Attendance Pension Benefit for caregivers of veterans of other wars. A guide to VA healthcare is also available. See, www.caregiver.va.gov for a checklist and a great tool for new Family Caregivers, questions to ask the doctor, and other information to help the caregiver stay organized with keeping track of all the things they must do.

RESCUE

RESCUE is a lifeline to help Caregivers learn about caregiving resources, and find self-help tools. RESCUE provides survival skills that will help you take better care of yourself and your loved one therefore if you are a caregiver of a veteran who had a stroke, visit the Resources and Education for Stroke Caregivers' Understanding and Empowerment (RESCUE) website.

Respite Care

Respite care is a temporary break for caregivers of the elderly, disabled, chronically or terminally ill, and it is an important resource for caregivers who can become easily stressed and suffer from caregiver burnout. Respite care is part of the Medicare Hospice Benefit and is also subsidized by many senior groups as well as private and government agencies. Respite care may be just the break the caregiver and loved one needs so discuss with your loved one's primary care about respite care, a sitter, hospice and medical coverage to see what options are available and which one works best for the caregiver and the loved one's needs.

Long-Term Care Insurance

A large percentage of people age 65 and over will need some type of long-term care services in their lifetime. Long-term care expenses are typically excluded from medical insurance plans. A long-term care insurance policy can help cover long-term care expenses you may experience during your retirement. Long-term care insurance is not something that everyone has, mainly because it isn't cheap. As a matter of fact, it is extremely costly, usually costing as much as $2,500 a month or close to $100,000.00 a year but if you can afford it, it sure would be nice to have especially for those who become physically and occupationally disabled with a cerebral or cognitive deficiency (i.e., dementia or Alzheimer's). The policy may allow physical and occupational therapists to cover the cost for a senior day-care facility, assisted living, rehabilitation or nursing home care that specializes in caring for cancer, dementia and Alzheimer's patients. Request a complimentary quote from a local licensed insurance agent to receive a no obligation and free consultation since it can be very complicated and expensive so avoid making a costly mistake by seeking the advice of a licensed insurance agent to decide if it is affordable, feasible, and meet your needs. Your health and financial security should determine whether you should purchase long-term care insurance or not. As with any insurance, the payouts will depend on the benefits and coverage you choose. Long-term care insurance may or may not cover some home care. Some policies permit family members to be paid, however, sometimes excluding those living within the same household. If your loved one has long-term care insurance, the insurance agent can clarify and explain the benefits, terms and conditions of that policy and provide any additional coverage needed.

Medicare does not offer any extended long-term care coverage. However, Medicaid offers long-term care for very low-income individuals only.

The insurance company's primary concern is that you can pay the premiums and that you do not exceed your total lifetime benefit. Also, make sure your policy includes an annual inflation adjustment rider which will adjust the daily benefit coverage by a set amount each year so that you do not buy a policy that could potentially double or triple in cost especially since you will be expected to pay the premium when you are retired or even if you're living on a reduced income. Always be mindful that if you stop paying any type of insurance policy, it could lapse, and you will lose your benefits and everything that you paid up to that point. Speak with an insurance agent when calculating how much you'll need to save for retirement to afford a long-term care insurance policy. If you are already retired or close to retirement make sure you have enough assets and that you can live off your retirement. If you are already struggling it will probably be a waste of your money and time to purchase long-term care insurance. Therefore, if you doubt you can afford a long-term care insurance policy through retirement you probably shouldn't purchase it. Whatever you purchase you'll have to live with it for many years to come, God willing, so choose a financially strong and stable company as well. Before you sign on the dotted line, ask the agent to provide you with the firm's latest financial strength grade from one of the major rating services such as Moody's or Standard & Poor's. An "A" rating or higher from Standard & Poor's or an "AA" ranking or better from Moody's Investor Service is a good indicator of financial strength and stability. The National Association of Insurance Commissioners (NAIC) recommends that you spend no more than 7% of your income on premiums.

If you are confused or need further assistance, consult a replicable financial planner for advice, one who can guide you through the decision making process to determine whether purchasing a long-term care insurance policy is beneficial and affordable for you. To locate a replicable fee-only financial planner (one that charges by the hour), visit the National Association of Personal Financial Advisors website. You can find free financial advice and help at http://www.free-financial-advice.net/.

When comparing policies, check the Better Business Bureau, your state insurance department, or the National

Association of Insurance Commissioners website for consumer complaints. Also check out an insurer's history of premium hikes from your state regulators. The fact that an insurer has imposed many price increases in the past, however, does not necessarily mean that it won't raise prices again; and ones that haven't raised rates still might do so therefore be careful, do your due diligence, and proceed with caution in choosing a long-term care insurance policy.

Many people do not acquire long term care insurance until they are 60 years old so unless you have a family history of a chronic disease (or Alzheimer's), and can afford the security (or luxury), you can wait and still be eligible for coverage, and probably pay less in the long run. Do not take my word for it, do your homework and due diligence when it comes to long-term care insurance because only you know what you want, what you can afford, and you are the only one that can be sure you're getting the coverage you need, and the best benefits for your buck.

Sometimes your best is not good enough and regardless of how hard you've worked, no matter what you have done to keep your loved one healthy, alive and at home, there may come a time when the burden is simply too much to handle and you may be forced to make the decision to move them into an outside long-term facility, and this is when long-term care insurance provides the most security, and is the most beneficial.

Estate Planning Checklist

People hate talking about death, but it is an important subject (a necessary evil, if you will) to discuss and a part of life. Therefore, if you refuse to talk about it, you should at least write down or express your wishes to your loved ones so that they will know your desires at the time of your death. However, if you really want to protect your loved one's interest or take care of your family you would do a Will or Trust. A Will can solve and eliminate all your problems and honor all your wishes. Although a trust can be an extremely useful estate planning tool, most people have no clue whether they need one or not or why they would need one at all. It is believed that only the rich and famous need a trust. Opening a trust can be very costly and complicated so if you do not have $100,000.00 or substantial assets in real estate it probably isn't worth it. A trust might be good for you if you have very explicit instructions regarding how to distribute your estate among heirs; for minimizing taxes; as well as protecting your estate from lawsuits and creditors.

A trust like anything else has its pros and cons. They can be broad, difficult and flexible. You should consult with an estate-planning attorney prior to setting up a trust. Anything not titled to the trust will have to go through probate.

Many cities hold free Wills & Trusts Workshops that you and your family can attend. The following questions may be helpful in your estate planning process:

- Have you appointed or authorized someone to handle financial matters for you in the event you became unable to?

- Do you know the gross value of your estate (including your house(s))? Do you have a Trust on a large estate?

- Do you have an executed Will?

- Have you reviewed your Will within the last three years?

- Does your Will name a guardian(s) (if you have minor child(ren))?

- Have you named executor(s) and/or trustee(s)?

- Do you have a permanent or long-term power of attorney?

- Have you made plans for your retirement?

- If you have specific wishes regarding your funeral, have you left instructions with your executor?

- Have you documented your wishes regarding organ donations? If so, do you have a donor card(s) stating that you have donated your body to a body donation program, and whether you're donating your full body, tissues, bone marrow, specific organs, etc., the contact information, and specific instructions not to embalm or autopsy at the time of your death?

- Do you have an Advanced Health Care Directive? Does it provide the names, addresses and telephone numbers of your designated agent(s)?

- Have you appointed an individual to distribute your personal property (including pets, if any) after your death?

- Do you have provisions in your Trust or Will for payment of estate taxes?

- Are there any changes in the gross value of your estate (the value of everything you own, not what you owe)?

- Have you recently married, remarried, divorced?

- Does your Will provide for children from a previous marriage(s)? Adopted children?

- If you have dependents with disabilities does your estate plan protect their interests?

- Do you have the correct type and right amount of life insurance?

- Have you inherited, bought or sold any property, stock or other assets?

- Have you moved between states?

- Have you considered making a planned gift to charity?

- Do you know what the tax and social security consequences would be for beneficiaries of your current Will?

- Does your Will protect potential beneficiaries who may face family breakdown or become bankrupt?

- Do you know what effect your death would have on your family financially or emotionally?

These are just a few of the more serious questions which most people simply do not know the answers to. You should consult with an estate planning attorney to determine if you need a trust and to gain knowledge about all the problems and pitfalls that you may face, including avoiding paying thousands of dollars to transfer everything you worked all your life for to your heirs as well as avoiding years of the probate process. Carefully note that if you do not properly designate who will inherit what, the state or city will make that decision for you. In most states, if you have not made plans, a judge of the Superior Court will decide who will raise your minor child(ren). If you become disabled, it could cost you and your family thousands of dollars just to have the right to take care of you and to direct your medical care. Educate yourself about "Joint Tenancy," which is the way that many married couples hold property which does not avoid probate. Holding title to property as "Joint Tenants" can cost thousands of dollars in capital gains taxes on the death of the first to die. Also, estate planning prepared before 2004 may not work now and it would be to your advantage to consult an estate planning attorney or attend a free seminar. If you plan properly, probate fees can cost you absolutely nothing – zero. Again, we know our birth date, but we do not know our expiration date, so get your house in order – think smart and think ahead, way ahead before it's too late. Life is no guarantee so be as prepared as you possibly can.

In those days Hezekiah was sick unto death and the prophet Isaiah, the son of Amoz came to him, and said unto him, Thus saith the LORD, set thine house in order; for thou shalt die, and not live. 2 Kings 20:1

Do the best you can do to keep your loved one encouraged, it will keep them from feeling hopeless and discouraged. You can keep yourself from being disheartened or dispirited as a caregiver by taking care of yourself as well as your loved one. Everyone is bound to have something, but we do not want the caregiver coming down with anything while caring for a loved one. The human body is resilient and amazing, so we should always challenge any ailment especially since we know that God is the maker and the creator of our bodies. He is a healer. He is a way-maker, a way out, miracle worker, and prayer has worked even when medicine has failed. God is the best medicine and sometimes He's the only medicine needed. God runs the ICU unit. God's care is more powerful than health care, medicine or doctors. We all know that God is bigger than all our problems and He cannot be outdone, and we are nothing without Him. He is so awesome, He was my caregiver – the caregiver's caregiver. I could not have done it without Him. Praise Him! Thank you, Lord!

I am the vine, ye are the branches: He that abideth in me, and I in him, the same bringeth forth much fruit: for without me ye can do nothing. John 15:5

The most magnificent reward that I take away from my caregiving experiences is that it brings you closer to God and makes you more aware of His presence. I was collapsing on my feet, but I never fell. I was stronger than I ever knew I could possibly be, all by the grace of God and I was able to run the race and endure it to the end because of Him. All Glory be to God! I take pride in finishing well. I want to thank Him for my journey up that steep, scary, harsh, and tough terrain and life of uncertainty. Thank you for being there to watch over me every step of the way, and thank you for picking me up when I was down. It wasn't easy, and I took a whipping but the more time I spent with God, the smoother the road became, and I began to experience more of His goodness, grace, mercy, and favor. I felt amazingly weak and just as amazingly strong. God made me realize that I was "down, but not out." When you are down you do not stay down, and when you get up, you have a testimony, it is a blesson and God's way of preparing and teaching you how to respond to others who are suffering. The Lord, does work in mysterious ways. He gave me all the courage and confidence I needed to get through each day and learn more about the gospel and the Holy Spirit along the way. I am Godspoiled! Thank you for such a rewarding experience and the blessons of possessing the care of giving spirit, dealing with life and death situations, and the understanding of how death ends a life but not a relationship, so however long we get to spend time with a loved one is precious, and a true blessing from God. Death leaves you feeling heartbroken and as though the hole in your heart will never heal but I knew that the love Rick and I shared and the memories we made were embedded in my heart like steel forever. In the end, God rewarded me with a life of staycation, every day being a vacation. He knew my walk before I even took the first step. I have an attitude of gratitude. Timing is everything. Seek Jesus and make time for God. I have seen many miracles, victories, and miraculous interventions.

As we become one with God, and take on His image, our goodness and principles does not come from us but from the God in us.

Also, if you don't know what your purpose is, start by working in your community, be a good neighbor, a good friend, health advocate, drug outreach coach, teen mentor, volunteer at a food bank, shelter, pet rescue, hospital, library, school, Big Sister, Big Brother, Boys & Girls Club, community recreation center volunteer – find your niche, your passion, God-given or hidden talent and chase it down, adopt a child, perform selfless acts of kindness and generosity, donate blood, be patient and loving, witness to others, love one another. Work at what makes you feel good, be blessed and be a blessing to others.

Chapter 9

Warning Signs

Rick's complications due to diabetes started when he was about 46 years old and by the time he was 50 it was all downhill from there and it all ended at 57. Looking back now to whether we had any warning signs before Rick got sick, and there were a lot of signs. When we walked the streets of the Virgin Islands, Rick literally could not keep up with me and we had to return to the hotel room to rest, take sitting breaks off and on throughout the day. Also, we often retired early in the evening. I encouraged him to spend time in the warm salty waters, he even had a couple of leg massages, and both gave him some relief but that salty water had me seeing spots, so I stayed on the beach but not in the water. In any event, I should have realized sooner that something was seriously wrong with Rick because I'm a walker and he was tiring so quickly that we would have to stop because his legs were aching so badly but since he was breathing perfectly fine I dismissed it to be nothing serious and concluded that he simply needed to drive less and walk more to strengthen his legs. He never complained about leg pain when bike riding or paddle boarding but when we went paddle boat riding, I did all the paddling but that's what I go for, For the exercise, and I thought he was just downright lazy. At home, we drove everywhere but when we traveled, we were very active and did a lot of walking and he did a lot of swimming and bike riding. I walked on my lunch hour, sometimes before work and after work too. I've always been a walker. I hated bike riding, but he loved it, so I obliged him, but I personally walked faithfully every day except I loved the bike path when we visited the Poconos Mountains in Pennsylvania during the fall.

On one occasion, all three of my kids were sitting at the kitchen table having a happy hour and sibling pow wow as I was cooking when Rick drove up.   After several long minutes had gone by, one of my sons said, "It sure is taking Rick a long time to come in the house, ma." I didn't think much of it and I joked, "Rick is just slow as molasses in January but maybe he's on the phone. He always moves like a snail." We laughed about him being too cool, calm and collected, not rushing for anyone. We all just poked fun at him taking forever to come into the house all the time but it when I think about, it was probably a sign that something was going terribly wrong with his vascular system, circulation and his legs. His mother was born with one kidney. His father died from a heart attack. The signs were there, especially genetically.   Rick went through it all, kidney failure, stroke and heart attack. He used to say that he had legs just like his grandmother, speaking about the appearance and shape but she also had a serious circulation and vascular problem. These were a lot of indicators that we ignored because we just did not know. You live, and you learn. This turned out to be a very costly lesson, Rick's life, at 57. I learned a lot and I wish I knew then, what I know now because I realize now that difficulty walking can even be an early sign or symptom of dementia as well.

Don't you realize that your body is the temple of the Holy Spirit, who lives in you and was given to you by God? You do not belong to yourself, for God bought you with a high price. So you must honor God with your body. 1 Corinthians 6:19-20

Wellness

Take care of your mental, physical, and emotional health; eat healthy now or be prepared to pay a team of doctors later. I'd rather take a bunch of vitamins now than take a bunch of pharmaceutical drugs later. With the proper diet and nutrition, we can teach our bodies to fight off diseases and perhaps learn a way to live without so many pharmaceutical drugs. You are what you eat and how you feel. How you feel is very important to your well-being. Emotional and mental health is just as crucial to your overall health and well-being as your physical health. Our emotional health is a critical factor that is ignored in our medical system. Good health requires focusing on the mind, body, spirit, food and wellness. Eat well, meditate, yoga, breathing exercises, painting, scrapbooking, and laughter is good for the soul so watch lots of comedies, and embrace your family and friends. Walking heals so make walking a priority in your daily lives. Work with your physician to figure out how everything can fit together to achieve happiness along with your best quality of life and optimal health. A start to taking control of your health is to have your physician devise a health measuring plan, so that if you are at high risk for diabetes, high blood pressure, heart attack, cancer or other autoimmune or chronic diseases, your doctor will be measuring any progress or decline to your health, and get you to the necessary specialists and/or team of doctors in a timely manner. In the meantime, remain in good spirits and if you must be a foodie, be a good foodie, and eat healthy.

Blessed are the pure in heart: for they shall see God. Matthew 5:8

In 2004 when Rick had his stroke, the hospitals back east where we lived then did not have a protocol in place to prevent or reverse a stroke. Today, there are infomercials on TV about how to recognize the symptoms of a stroke, on the internet, and all hospitals have a protocol in place and signs posted throughout the hospital and in the emergency room, so be cautious, aware of your vital signs, and take care of your health and spirit.

A merry heart doeth good [like] a medicine: but a broken spirit drieth the bones. Proverbs 17:22

Meditation and yoga alone can create the health you desire, and we can also create the health we desire. Your health must matter to you because if you do not care about you, why should anyone else? Your health can change in an instant, in a blink of an eye. You, literally, are what you eat and your diet, for the most part, determines how well you feel. You must take care of your health now to avoid health issues or complications later. When it comes to eating, everything is in moderation and everything should be pleasant to your taste buds. Remove all processed foods from your diet. One good way to remove processed food from your diet altogether is to shop the outside aisles at the grocery store where you will find your fresh meats, juices, dairy, fruits and vegetables. If you don't already know, you will be pleasantly surprised to learn how fruits, vegetables, beans, weeds, seeds and herbs can prevent, fight against, support, reduce risks, manage, support and regulate certain medical conditions and chronic diseases.

I am not a doctor so please take everything with care and consult your physician or an expert in botanical medicine before making any changes to your medication or diet. However, animal studies suggest that fruits and vegetables might help humans to reduce chronic illnesses, but human studies haven't been conducted to support many of these theories. To be honest, botanical medicine is not a bad thing.

Holistic health has been used for thousands of years in ancient healing practices and is just beginning to be recognized in mainstream medical practice as a broad view of patient care.

Avoid nostrums and patent medicines. The habitual use of any drug is harmful. The most eminent physicians all now agree that very few drugs have any real curative value. The essential thing is right habits of life. John Harvey Kellogg

Taking control of your health is a great start to caring about you. "If you do not take care of you, you will not be able to take care of anyone else." Make healthy families and communities by becoming a health advocate for you, your family, friends and community.

And they cast out many demons, and anointed with oil many who were sick, and healed them. Mark 6:13

The fact is that "no pharmaceutical drug is without side effects," or "without harm," and that's the most unfortunate thing about prescription drugs since while you are treating one illness, you could be creating another one. Some healthier staples may also have cautions, warnings and/or side effects which are not listed or that you are not even made aware of. As my dad used to say, "Too much of anything isn't good for you," so to be on the safe side, do everything in moderation, including over-the-counter drugs. Also, be sure to read the side effects and warnings about any over-the-counter and prescription medications that you take.

Now faith is the substance of things hoped for, the evidence of things not seen. Hebrews 11:1

Chapter 10

Body and Organ Donor Awareness

Hundreds of thousands of Americans require a transplant and the need for organ donors has never been greater. Kidneys, liver, kidney/pancreas, lung, pancreas, and the intestines are organs needed for transplants. If you ever wanted to help someone else live, you can become a living or deceased donor. Living donors have the power to not only improve a patient's quality of life, rather it can save a person's life while you are still alive. Due to the rise in obesity and diabetes, the demand for kidneys cannot be met through deceased donations alone. Liver disease is increasing and living liver transplants can be a viable option for some patients. The liver regenerates very fast, and within three months the donor's liver function should be back to normal. I am a full-body donor and I was going to donate a kidney to my husband, but he did not want to have a kidney transplant. He said he felt bad enough as it was, and he was not willing to go through the recovery process and the surgery was a 50/50 risk of life and death. If you consider being a live or deceased organ and tissue donor you could save one or several lives. By becoming an organ donor, you can save the lives of as many as eight people and improve the lives of dozens who are desperately in need of an organ transplant. I can only imagine the reward one must feel when donating an organ, being so selfless and so generous, to give a part of themselves to save another's life and we can only imagine how blessed the recipient must feel when they receive the gift of life.

Unfortunately, many Americans die because they are unable to get an organ donation. My husband eventually died from kidney disease also.

This is my commandment, that you love one another as I have loved you. Greater love has no one than this, that someone lay down his life for his friends. John 15:12-13

Whether you are interested or not in being an organ donor, visit the website: "activebeat.com" to learn why organ donation is so incredibly important and you will no longer be confused or believe the myths you have heard about organ donation. Educate yourself about organ donation by contacting your local university to inquire about their full-body, organ and tissue programs. You can also visit www.DMV.org/organdonor; and when at the DMV, select "Yes" to organ donation and get a donor card, if available when you apply or renew your driver's license; register with any county or state organ donor registry, contact a Living Bank, or contact your local universities to inquire about their organ donor programs. I commend the donors who have already saved lives and the registered donors who have hopes of giving the gift of life and interested in saving and improving lives. I support the researchers, innovators, advocates, doctors, scientist, and other medical professionals working to reduce the number of people waiting for vital organ transplants and I will continue to pray to expand the availability of organs for transplants, and more donors for the many recipients needing an organ transplant. With kidney transplants if you are not a match for a family member or friend whom you wish to donate to, you may be a match for another kidney transplant recipient and another donor could be a match for you—win, win situation. Please consider being a true lifesaver by giving the true gift of life.

About the Authoress

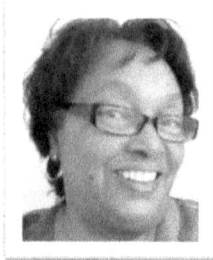

The authoress, Jean Renee Porter has books under the name of Jean Renee Johnson as well. She is a Washington, DC native, and most of her life she lived in the DMW (Washington DC, Maryland and Virginia). Ms. Porter grew up in northeast and northwest Washington, DC and is proud to say that she is a product of the DC Public School System. She graduated from Theodore Roosevelt Senior High School, attended Strayer University and the U.S. Department of Agriculture Graduate School. Ms. Porter is now a retired legal assistant and widow, living a life of staycation, every day being a vacation in beautiful and sunny Southern California where people pay to visit. She lives in Desert Hot Springs (DHS), "California's Spa City" as it is known for its naturally occurring water aquifers and home to the country's largest collection of hot mineral springs that contributes to the city's award-winning drinking water and the many boutique spas and resorts. It is beautifully situated between the San Bernardino National Forest, Joshua Tree National Park, and Mount Jacinto State Park, therefore offering lots of scenic views and outdoor recreation as well as the Cabot's Pueblo Museum, a historical, cultural and educational Native American museum, displaying a variety of artifacts and attractions enjoyed by locals and visitors. Palm Springs, the President's playground, the celebrities' oasis and getaway, and the Cabazon shopping outlets are just a short drive from Desert Hot Springs as is easy access to San Diego and Los Angeles.

Ms. Porter has been writing since she was seven years old and credits her parents and the village that raised her for their

267

motivation, including ninth grade music teacher, Roberta Flack; business teacher, Mrs. Dorothy Moorman; typing teacher, Mrs. Simms; shorthand teacher, B. K. Williams. They all inspired, mentored, supported, took a special interest in her at a very young age, and encouraged her to write and follow her dreams.

Her legal career actually began at 14 years old when she worked as a summer aide for the Department of Agriculture, Office of the General Counsel, Rural Electrification Division. At 16, she was an ambitious teenage mom, student and summer office assistant. Although she was a young mom, she still graduated from high school on time and after graduation she became a civil service GS-2 employee and was promoted to a GS3-4 and 5, within two years. She also attended Strayer College and the Department of Agriculture Graduate School. Ms. Porter was very fortunate to be a young adult in an era where employers reimbursed employees if they maintained a good grade point average in college. Ms. Porter has taken advantage of every opportunity that comes her way to improve on her life, knowledge, good leadership and social skills. She strongly believes that God communicates with us through opportunities and challenges to see how we handle them or don't handle them. She believes in miracles and God's miraculous interventions, divine placement and stepping into that moment of opportunity.

After three years, she left the Agriculture Department to pursue opportunities in the private sector. She worked for consultants, a public relations firm, numerous DC law firms, a nonprofit organization (the Drug Abuse Council, during President Carter's term was about fighting the war on drugs in the 70s as well as the legalization and decriminalization of marijuana. We also researched methadone to see how it

could be used to ween people off heroin, the effects it would
have on their body long-term and how methadone could be
used for palliative care to reduce pain in terminally ill
patients which it is being used today especially with
terminally ill pancreatic patients.)   At the Drug Abuse
Council, she worked as a Legal Assistant to the staff Legal
Counsel.   She also worked at the Aspen Institute for
Humanistic Studies, a roundtable think-tank organization as
an Executive Secretary to the Vice President. She and her
family traveled to Aspen, Colorado, an unforgettable
experience for her and her sons).   In the late 70's, she
cherishes meeting the Carter's and having her picture taken
with Rosalyn Carter and considers it to be the most
memorable experience in her life. Ms. Porter also worked
closely with the National Organization for the Reform of
Marijuana Laws (NORML) on the legalization and
decriminalization of marijuana. For close to four decades,
she worked at various law firms in Washington, DC as a
Legal Secretary, Legal Assistant, and Freelance Legal
Assistant. Ms. Porter also worked for a public relations firm,
Hager Sharp and Abramson in DC. Her duties included
working with the late Mayor Marion Barry's office and
various DC public high schools introducing seniors to the
hospitality and tourism industry in Washington, DC. Being
a native Washingtonian, it gave her great honor to be able to
mentor students from the high school where she was an
alumnus as well as many other high schools in the DC area.

When asked about her legal experiences, she said, "I dislike
lawyers a whole lot because all they care about the dollar
bill, debating and arguing about any and everything, and
although they may not win in the court room or even ever

step foot in a court room, and although they may not always
be right, they are never wrong. They are the big boss, so it
is their way or no way. Lawyers have no filter, they want
what they want when they want it. They even think planes
fly when they want them to fly. They have big egos and are
difficult people to work with. It was like a bad marriage,
they were impatient, overbearing, too demanding,
nitpickers, never wrong, refused to agree to disagree,
coldhearted, no love whatsoever, and worst of all, they had
no problem with making and changing rules as they went
along; inflicting insults, firing and threatening employees'
jobs without an ounce of remorse. Working for such
difficult people and trying to be a team player was hard. The
women partners were way worse than the men if you can
imagine that. What I liked the most about the legal field was
the knowledge I had to have to navigate myself through the
daily challenges; the constant fires I had to put out; the level
of productivity and expectation; pay and bonuses;
professionalism, and conscientiousness. Money motivated
me, and they paid and treated me well. Lawyers taught me
as a teen that 'errors slow down production' and that has
been a great asset to my life, so despite how much I dislike
them, I really love legal, and I appreciate the opportunities,
blessons, and all the doors that God opened for me because
I went through many doors and working with lawyers
afforded me a great break in life with the demand being so
great for someone with my abilities, qualifications and years
of experience. I learned a lot since there was very little room
for errors which gave me the opportunity to perfect my
writing craft, proofing and editing skills over the years. My
parents had already instilled in me good work ethics, but
lawyers made a professional and a perfectionist out of me.
They helped me prove to me, myself and I, and they gave me
the confidence that I could take anywhere. I am thankful and
they all know it, even the ones I constantly challenged on the
job and/or complained about, and the most important thing

is that we agreed to disagree, remained professional associates, acquaintances, or friends over the years because no matter what, I received excellent evaluations, raises and bonuses, I just believed in standing up for what I believed in. In the end, all I had to do was go to work, do my job and do it well, and I had them eating out the palm of my hands. My parents raised me to have tough skin to survive in this world, 'sticks and stones may break my bones, but words should never hurt me,' which was also a valuable blesson. I just wish they had taught me to bite my tongue a little more because I way too outspoken and always taking up for others as well."

Ms. Porter is a spiritually gifted life coach, speaker and positive person with a very giving nature. The gift to write has given her the opportunity to freely express herself, and although she may not be rich financially she's very rich in love, emotions, thoughts and knowledge. She has an attitude of gratitude. Writing is not only a gift it is a God-given talent, it's the most joyful part of her life, and she finds writing to be very therapeutic – it relaxes her mind, body, and spirit, as well as promotes wellness.

Ms. Porter's children and grandchildren are her world. They keep her grounded, motivated, upbeat and young spirited. Even at the age of 65 she loves to jump rope and dance and she thanks God for the ability to do so even with arthritis in her ankle, foot, wrist, knee and sciatica nerve. She says it works like a charm every single time.

When she was a teen, she danced on a local television show in Washington, DC, Channel 14 (WOOK) Teenarama Dance Party hosted by Bob King in the late 60s through the early 70s and she was the youngest regular dancing on the show during that time. She was very mature for her age, she was considered an old soul by the elders in the family, older neighbors, and her mother said she was 10 when she was born.

She is not only an authoress she is also a poet and lyricist. Over the years, she has had contract offers with recording studios in Hollywood and Nashville however she had to decline their offers due to money and time constraints and of course, caregiving responsibilities. Many of her poems are published in anthologies that are read all over the world. Ms. Porter has written over 400 poems/lyrics. She basically writes poetry for fun, therapy and relaxation. Writing also puts her in a great mind space to connect with and touch the lives of others.

Ms. Porter has many accomplishments, including creating new words that she hopes to see in the dictionary one day in the not-to-distant future. The use of the word will determine the timing of its publication. Ms. Porter is the self-published authoress of the following books, articles, poems, words, and songs:

Books
- *Every Ending Has a New Beginning*, published 2002, nine short stories about relationships inspired by actual experiences. (Not a spiritual book.)

- *A Positive Influence Poetry Collection: Simply Godly*, published in 2003, spiritual poems thanking God.

- *Inside DC Law Firms: The Real Deal (From A Secretary's Perspective)*, published 2005, about law firm experiences, inspired by actual experiences.

- *Malcolm: The Guinea Pig King*, published 2017, children's book about a child with asthma and allergies who really wanted a pet, so he settled for a guinea pig who doesn't have the same allergens and dander like dogs and cats have.

- *Paige and Her Nine Dogs*, published 2017, children's book about an only child with nine dogs who are more like her siblings. Paige receives the best 5th birthday gift most children can only dream about, but it meant leaving all her dogs behind.

- *Faith-lift Quotes*, published June 2017, daily faith-lifts and inspirational quotes.

- *The Care of Giving (Family-In-Home Caregiving)*, published December 2017 is about in-home caregiving from beginning to end and was inspired by actual experiences. It expresses how the authoress felt, what she went through, how she survived it, and some tools she learned along the way when she was a health advocate, intensive, progressive and proactive caregiver, 24-7 to her husband for seven years, who was a diabetic with complications, including glaucoma, plus he was among the few men to have a lump removed from his breast to prevent breast cancer; he was a heart attack and stroke survivor, on dialysis, wheelchair bound, bedridden and dementia. Ms. Porter became a certified peritoneal dialysis technician so that her husband could do dialysis at home.

- *Our Body, His Temple (God's Free Health and Wellness Plan)* is a compilation of vegetables, fruits, beans, nuts, spices, vitamins, seeds, and weeds, and their health benefits relative to chronic diseases and how our health and what we eat also relates to the

Bible. It is a work in progress of years of research and written in hopes of saving lives, curing and preventing chronic diseases through better health choices, diet and nutrition, and perhaps help us to figure out how to live without pharmaceutical drugs. It is the authoress' belief that by the grace of God, along with proper diet, nutrition and exercise, we can teach our bodies to fight off diseases. Publication, December 2017.

Articles
- *Self-Publishing, Writinghood,* May 20, 2009
- *Help to Prevent a Stroke by Checking Your Pulse, HealthMad,* May 21, 2009
- *What is LDL and HDL Cholesterol? HealthMad,* May 21, 2009
- *Rusted Kitchen Utensils, Gomestic,* June 16, 2009
- *Thunderstorm Safety, Gomestic,* June 16, 2009
- *Kidney Disease and Antiperspirants,* HealthMad, July 31, 2009
- *Inner Peace, Socyberty,* December 24, 2010
- *How to Deter Burglars, unpublished*
- *Telling the Truth, unpublished*
- *Weak Owner and Protective Dog = Bad Combo, unpublished*

Songs
- Home
- So Others Will Survive (a tribute to the U.S. troops), published by Song Partners in Sarasota, Florida

Poems

- So Others Will Survive (published in Best Poems and Poets of 2003 and Our 100 Most Famous Poets, The Brief Chronicles of Our Time.

- Finding Peace (featured in *Best Poems and Poets of 2002*).

- Stay Strong (published in *On Gossamer Wings*) were written when she was trying to find peace within herself after the events of September 11th.

- It's Time (featured in *Letters from the Soul*) is a poem about acknowledging love.

- Flowers is a very touching poem about giving a person their flowers before it's too late or while they're living and is published in *Eternal Portraits* and a special CD poetry collection, *The Sound of Music*.

- Too Young to Let Go, is a poem to encourage parents not to give up on their young children and is published in London, U.K., and featured in *Theatre of the Minds*.

- Only God Can (written as she tried to wrap her mind around the Paris Planned Parenthood and the San Bernardino, California senseless bombings.

Words

- Godspoiled - to be blessed and favored by God; personal praise to God.

- Copeless – no hope; no faith; unable to move forward.

Awards and Accomplishments
- Nominated Poet of the Year
- Editor's Choice Awards for her Outstanding Accomplishments in Poetry
- Poet of the Year Medallion and the Shakespeare Trophy of Excellence
- Certificate of Achievement for Outstanding Achievement in Poetry for exclusive publication by the Famous Poets Society
- Inducted as an International Poet of Merit
- Honored Member of the International Society of Poets
- Who's Who in Poetry, 2005, 2007.

References

AARP Caregiving Resource Center, www.aarp.org/caregiving.

Ferguson, Dr. Elaine, "Super Healing: Engaging Your Mind, Body, and Spirit to Create Optimal Health and Well-being," October 1, 2013.

New King James Bible via
https://www.biblegateway.com/passage/?search=

New King James Version (NKJV), The Lord's Prayer, Matthew 6:7-15.

Kubler-Ross, Elisabeth, Quotes, https://www.goodreads.com/author/quotes/1506.Elisabeth_K_bler_Ross

Kubler-Ross, Elisabeth, On Death and Dying, June 9, 1977.

New Living Translation Bible

http://www.alz.org/10-signs-symptoms-alzheimers-dementia.asp

https://www.alz.org/documents_custom/2016-facts-and-figures.pdf

http://www.alz.org/alzheimers_disease_causes_risk_factors.asp

https://www.alz.org/downloads/facts_figures_2012.pdf

http://www.aspentimes.com/news/15936744-113/80-year-old-earns-aspens-100-day-skiing-pin

www.care.com

www.caregiver.va.gov

www.caregiving.com

http://www.caregiver.va.gov/toolbox/index.asp#sthash.h3TleLjs.dpuf

http://www.cbsnews.com/news/pat-summitts-death-what-to-know-about-early-onset-alzheimers/

www.familyofavet.com/va.caregiver_program

http://idrp.pbrc.edu/faq.htm

http://money.cnn.com/retirement/guide/ or
Retirementliving_healthcare.moneymag/index13.htm, Long-term care insurance.

http://my.clevelandclinic.org/health/transcripts/1528_young-onset-dementias

http://www.npr.org/sections/thetwo-way/2014/06/02/318238155/91-year-old-woman-breaks-marathon-record

http://www.ocala.com/article/20130331/ARTICLES/130339991?p=1&tc=pg&tc=ar

https://www.sciencedaily.com/releases/2016/06/160616071933.htm

www.supportnetwork.heart.org

http://www.wsj.com/articles/at-95-a-lifelong-skiier-says-the-source-of-his-vitality-is-his-workout-1448899633

https://www.biblegateway.com/passage/?search=2+Corinthians+5&version=NLT

http://www.whatchristianswanttoknow.com/bible-verses-for-encouragement-20-great-scripture-quotes/#ixzz4dcrgDgiY